T0073147

LIVING WITH COVID-19

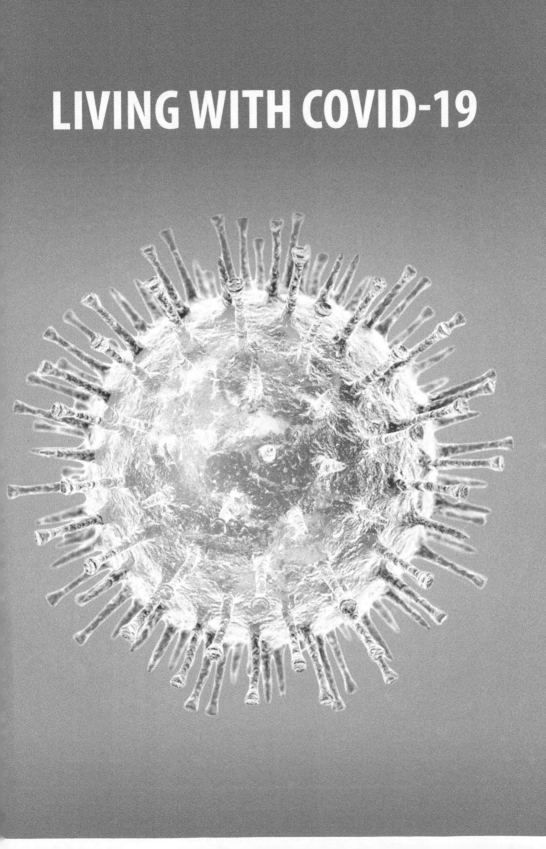

LIVING WITH COVID-19

Economics, Ethics, and Environmental Issues

edited by

Chaudhery Mustansar Hussain
Gustavo Marques da Costa

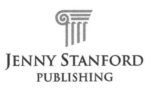

JENNY STANFORD
PUBLISHING

Published by

Jenny Stanford Publishing Pte. Ltd.
Level 34, Centennial Tower
3 Temasek Avenue
Singapore 039190

Email: editorial@jennystanford.com
Web: www.jennystanford.com

British Library Cataloguing-in-Publication Data
A catalogue record for this book is available from the British Library.

Living with COVID-19: Economics, Ethics, and Environmental Issues

Copyright © 2022 Jenny Stanford Publishing Pte. Ltd.

ISBN 978-981-4877-78-7 (Hardcover)
ISBN 978-1-003-16828-7 (eBook)

Contents

Preface

At the end of 2019, the world came across a virus, SARS-CoV-2. This new coronavirus causes a disease classified as COVID-19. The virus is highly transmissible and causes an acute respiratory syndrome that ranges from mild symptoms in about 80% cases to very severe symptoms with respiratory failure in 5% to 10% cases. The World Health Organization has declared the outbreak of COVID-19 to be a pandemic and classified it as a high global risk. Among the risks, we have risk of exposure and, in this way, we can assess occupational exposure to waste from health services. Human health risk assessment is a process of gathering and analyzing environmental and health information, using specific techniques to support decision-making, and executing, systematically, actions and articulation within and between sectors to promote health, improving the social and living conditions of the populations. The risk assessment for COVID-19 needs to consider and document all relevant information available at the time of the assessment. The government and funding agencies need to constantly invest in research involving treatments, vaccines, diagnosis, pathogenesis and natural history of the disease, disease burden, health care, prevention, and control in the COVID-19 area. This book addresses in detail the challenges posed by the virus and presents up-to-date knowledge on the economics, ethics, and environmental issues of COVID-19.

The book is divided into 12 chapters involving topics such as behavior of the COVID-19 virus in the environment; protective equipments for personnel dealing with it; and ethical, economic, and legal issues related to it. The book is important because it contributes significantly to the development of scientific and technological support required to confront and understand COVID-19 and its consequences. It is a good source of knowledge for advanced undergraduate and graduate students and provides guidelines for their studies. In addition, the book will be of significant interest to researchers and scientists working on the basic issues related to COVID-19, and due to its multidisciplinary nature, it will prove to be a good reference book for all those who are involved and interested in the challenges and discoveries of new security risks of COVID-19 as well as advancements in different areas related to the virus.

We are thankful to all chapter authors, who are subject experts from academia and industry, for their enthusiastic efforts in bringing out this book. We also extend special thanks to the team at Jenny Stanford Publishing for their support in publishing it. We are sure it will turn out to be a milestone in this subject.

Chaudhery Mustansar Hussain
Gustavo Marques da Costa
Summer 2021

Chapter 1

COVID-19 in the Environment

Gabriela Zimmermann Prado Rodrigues,
Aline Belem Machado, Juliana Machado Kayser,
Günther Gehlen, and Daiane Bolzan Berlese

Feevale University, ERS-239, 2755, 93525-075, Novo Hamburgo,
Rio Grande do Sul, Brazil
gabizpr@gmail.com, linebmachado@hotmail.com, ju.kayser@hotmail.com,
guntherg@feevale.br, daianeb@feevale.br

1.1 Definition and Origin of COVID-19

The first outbreaks of the current pandemic were reported in December 2019, among patients who were hospitalized and initially diagnosed with pneumonia. Subsequently, it was observed that these individuals had epidemiological links with the wholesale market for wet animals and seafood in Wuhan, Hubei Province, China [1]. The first atypical case of pneumonia recognized as the result of contamination by a new coronavirus was confirmed by the World Health Organization (WHO) on December 31, 2019 [2], and 26 days later, 2033 cases and 56 deaths had already been confirmed [3]. As of January 21, 2021, the virus had infected 95,321,880 people and caused 2,058,226 deaths across the world.

Living with COVID-19: Economics, Ethics, and Environmental Issues
Edited by Chaudhery Mustansar Hussain and Gustavo Marques da Costa
Copyright © 2022 Jenny Stanford Publishing Pte. Ltd.
ISBN 978-981-4877-78-7 (Hardcover), 978-1-003-16828-7 (eBook)
www.jennystanford.com

Severe acute respiratory syndrome (SARS) is caused by the new coronavirus 2 (SARS-CoV-2)—a virus classified as a group 2B β CoV, one that has at least some similarity in the genetic sequence to SARS-CoV-1 [4], which was responsible for the zoonosis that originated in China and caused 8903 cases of infection in 2002 and 2003 [5]. The clinical spectrum of SARS-CoV-2 pneumonia varies from mild to severe, and further details will be discussed in the following topics of this chapter.

1.2 Transmission of COVID-19

The new coronavirus 2, as well as the other existing coronaviruses, belong to the family Coronaviridae (subfamily Coronavirinae) and are found in both humans and animals. Structurally, it consists of a single-stranded RNA surrounded by a fat-coated substance. They are considered enveloped viruses, and the longest among RNA viruses [6, 4], with a size ranging from 80 nm to 120 nm and five single-stranded positive-sense RNA genomes, between 26.2 and 31.7 kb in length [6]. The symptoms caused range from the common cold to the more extreme respiratory, enteric, liver, and neurological symptoms [7], including inflammatory-based infections [8].

Viral entry depends on a good virus-host cell interaction. The infection is initiated by the interaction of the viral particle with specific proteins on the cell surface [6]. Enveloped viruses need to fuse their envelope with the host cell membrane to deliver their nucleocapsid to the target cell, and in the case of coronavirus 2, the spike protein acts by mediating in this receptor binding as well as in the membrane fusion [6]. This protein is responsible for the denomination of "crown" that the virus has received—it is grouped on the surface of the virus [6]. But it should be noted that viruses, in general, exploit their host cells to first express viral genes, then optimize the cell environment, and then fully activate the viral replication program [9].

To infect a new host, coronaviruses need to adapt to the host's receptor (mutation or recombination); SARS-CoV, for example, appeared in live animal markets, also in China, in 2002, and these animals were recognized as the intermediate hosts during the jump in the species [6]. In the specific case of coronavirus 2, which, as already mentioned, is a betacoronavirus, the main receptor is the angiotensin-converting enzyme 2 (ACE2) [6], which is a type I integral membrane protein, expressed in the lung tissue and responsible for the hydrolysis of angiotensin II [6]. But it is already known that the coronavirus is capable of exploring uncountable other cell-surface molecules in order to infect the cell, as is the case of calcium-dependent lectins [6].

Briefly, SARS-CoV and SARS-CoV-2 bind with and negatively regulate ACE2 in the cell [10], which basically regulates vasoconstrictor and proinflammatory effects through the p38 protein [11]. Therefore, the loss of ACE2 activity after viral entry into the cell can result in uncontrolled inflammation [12]. Since the way of entering the cell is relatively simple, it should be emphasized that these infectious agents can spread from their natural reservoir to a susceptible host through different pathways [13] which will be addressed later in this chapter.

Infected people transmit the viral particles whenever they speak, sneeze, or cough, and such particles are encapsulated in mucus globules, saliva, and water, and their destinations depend on their respective sizes [13]. Larger droplets tend to fall before evaporation, while smaller particles evaporate more quickly as aerosols, remaining in the air and moving further away than droplets [13–15]. Therefore, respiratory particles can be differentiated into droplets and aerosols on the basis of the particle size [16]. The WHO [17] considers particles larger than 5 μm as droplets and particles smaller than 5 μm as aerosols.

Consequently, aerosols pose a greater risk of spreading COVID-19, although over long distances or over time virus dilution and inactivation may occur [18]. In general, aerosols are also responsible for most infections in the alveolar tissues of the lower respiratory tract, precisely because of their small size, while the larger droplets are trapped in the upper airways [19]. Regardless of the particle size, the risk of transmission of the virus in social contacts is high, and for this reason, the measure adopted worldwide as a way of containing the rapid spread of the pandemic is social distance.

The risks are similar to those of any other infectious disease transmitted by any other respiratory virus or other sources. For example, surgery and medical procedures, tap water, and flushing also generate aerosols that may contain the pathogen [13], just as physical contact between an infected individual and a possible susceptible host or indirect contact with infectious secretions can also cause the transmission of the pathogens by contact [20]. In addition, in the specific case of COVID-19, Ong et al. [21] analyzed the exhausts of air in a hospital room with patients with the disease. The result was positive, suggesting that small aerosols loaded with viruses could be displaced by the airflow.

Wang and colleagues [22] investigated the fecal contamination of 205 COVID-19 positive patients in China and reported viral load in 29% of the stool samples. Consequently, the virus has been reported in sewage waters in several countries [23–25]. A recent study also indicated that the virus remains on plastic and steel surfaces for up to 72 hours, in small but still viable amounts [26], indicating that transmission via contaminated surfaces is also possible in the case of COVID-19.

When mucus or saliva is ejected from an infected person, its trajectory is determined mainly by the size of the droplets and the airflow patterns that govern the movement paths [27]. For this reason, scenarios such as field hospitals and other health centers specialized in the treatment of COVID-19 are high-risk environments for infection—due to the continuous and cross flow of air [13].

Under normal conditions, a distance of 2 m is considered "safe" to prevent the transmission of contaminated particles from the infected person to the possible host. However, like any pandemic, new studies are constantly changing theories built at the beginning of the problem. For example, Loh et al. [28] demonstrated that droplets carrying pathogens can travel about 7–8 m in a sneeze and about 2 m during coughing, regardless of the particle size.

Numerous environmental factors, in addition to the air direction, as already mentioned, can interfere with the viral load and consequently the degree of infection of the disease, and Jayaweera et al. [13] bring together a large number of these factors in their study. Ambient temperatures of 22°C–25°C associated with relative humidity <20% or >80%, for example, enable higher rates of SARS-CoV survival on smooth surfaces, simulating typical air-conditioning environments [29]. In contrast, temperatures of 38°C with relative humidity >95%, simulating tropical climates, demonstrate loss of viability of SARS-CoV [29]. Rapid and unexpected changes in temperature, simulating hot and cold days, resulted in an increase in SARS-CoV cases [30].

However, in conditions outside the laboratory, these rules are not always repeated. Brazil, for example, reported the first case of COVID-19 in mid-February 2020 and is currently in the third position in the ranking of countries with the highest number of cases, behind only the United States and India. It should be noted that in Brazil, the highest incidence in the number of cases is found in regions where the climate is typically tropical, with high temperatures, indicating that probably the virus has undergone an adaptation or alteration in its genetic material, resulting in an increase in its virulence. So, different populations around the world have adopted different habits to reduce the spread of the virus, especially the population groups that need to continue with their work activities, which will be addressed in the following sections of this chapter.

1.3 Environmental Impacts

The COVID-19 pandemic has caused countless problems worldwide, such as health issues, economic crisis [30], starvation, and unemployment [31]. The environment was also impacted by this virus and, as the other problems mentioned above, will probably last for an unevaluable period.

The viruses could enter the environment from affected people, symptomatic or asymptomatic, through their excreta [32]. SARS-CoV-2 RNA was detected in water systems in India [33], Australia [23], Japan [24], and Italy [25]. These studies demonstrated the environmental pollution caused by COVID-19 and the anthropogenic effects in the aquatic systems.

Although fecal-oral transmission is not yet proven and well established [34], it can be a threat to the environment [35]. The capacity of SARS-CoV-2 to spread in the environment by sewage sludge and wastewater must be taken into consideration. SARS-CoV-2 RNA was found in different water systems worldwide [33]. Wastewater-based epidemiology is being performed to monitor the prevalence of SARS-CoV-2 among the population [23]. These studies can also demonstrate the environmental impact that coronavirus is causing in different aquatic systems.

When the WHO declared COVID-19 as a pandemic and the virus was spreading rapidly, cities around the world started the lockdown. In Wuhan city, China, the epicenter of the pandemic, 200 tons of clinical trash was produced by 11 million people in just 1 day (February, 24, 2020), which was four times over the capacity the dedicated facility could incinerate in a day [36].

Another worldwide issue related to waste disposal is the use of masks, gloves, and hand sanitizers. As the pandemic grew, there grew a necessity for personal protective equipment (PPE) as a way to prevent both health-care workers and the population in general [37] from getting infected (symptomatic or asymptomatic), leading to the generation of huge amounts medical waste contaminated with the virus [38] around the world, a matter of huge concern.

A mask can be worn no longer than 1 day, and used masks and empty bottles of hand sanitizers are being discarded in huge amounts by the population, sometimes erroneously, and ending up in the environment [36]. For the world population of 7.8 billion, it is estimated that 129 billion face masks and 65 billion gloves are being used per month. Used gloves and masks are being found in public spaces, which will probably remain in the environment for decades, resulting in the contamination of the biota and biological systems [39].

Other indirect negative effects caused by the pandemic were the suspension of recycling programs in the United States due to the risk of contamination by the recyclable trash and the restriction of sustainable waste management in European countries. For example, Italy prohibited infected residents from sorting their waste. The lockdown imposed by the authorities has increased online ordering, such as for food, which has resulted in an increase in the domestic waste as well [40].

The waste generated during the pandemic, such as plastics and drugs, particularly waster that is not biodegradable, will persist for a longer period in wastewater [41].

Though COVID-19 caused and will continue causing negative impacts on the environment, positive impacts have also occurred during the pandemic, which can be described as good, such as a reduction in the environmental noise, cleaner beaches, and a decrease in the air pollution [40].

The necessity and obligation of social distancing in many different countries have caused the absence of tourists on beaches, which resulted in cleaner waters around the world, such as in Mexico, Spain, and Ecuador. Also, because of the same distancing measures imposed by the authorities to prevent the spread of the virus, many changes occurred in the daily activities, such as the decreased use of private and public transportation and the halt of commercial activities, resulting in a considerable reduction in the noise level worldwide [40].

When the outbreak of COVID-19 epidemic occurred in China, the country's major industries operated at lower levels than usual. The use of coal and crude oil also decreased during the lockdown. These measures all together resulted in a CO_2 emission reduction of 25% or more, which means that carbon emissions were reduced by around 1 million tons in 2020, compared to the emissions in the same time period of 2019, which is equal to 6% of the global emission [42].

Nitrogen dioxide (NO_2) gas is harmful to our health. It can corrode the lung tissue, and exposure to high concentrations can cause respiratory symptoms. The sources of this gas are oil, coal, and natural gas combustion and vehicular exhaust [42]. The European Space Agency (ESA) and the National Aeronautics and Space Administration released satellite images of air pollution from around the world [43]. These agencies estimated a decrease of around 30% in NO_2 gas during the lockdown period of the country under analysis (Italy, Spain, France, China, and the United States).

The ESA reported a decrease of around 40% in sulfur dioxide (SO_2) gas during the pandemic. Sulfur dioxide can be produced by natural processes, such as volcanoes, but also from anthropogenic sources, such as power plants burning fossil fuels [44]. The decrease in air pollutants emphasizes the positive impacts of the COVID-19 pandemic. However, this impact is temporary because once the industrial activity returns to its normal level, the concentration of air pollutants will increase to the prepandemic levels.

Therefore, the COVID-19 pandemic has had both negative and positive impacts on the environment. Unfortunately, the positive impacts will last for a shorter time than the negative ones—it is still uncertain how long the negative impacts will last and how bad they will be for the environment in general.

1.4 Prevention of COVID-19

COVID-19 is considered a global threat, and it has been the cause of deaths of thousands of people around the world [45]. Government agencies have adopted preventive measures with the aim of limiting the global spread of the virus on the basis of the current scientific knowledge [46]. However, one of the challenges is to achieve social commitment not only in the public health sector but in all areas that encompass society [47].

First of all, the population should be well informed about the virus and how to prevent contamination [45, 48]. The authorities have to use different means of communication to provide and diffuse information in a timely and accurate manner to build trust and avoid panic [48]. At the beginning of the pandemic, most of the countries elaborated strategies to limit the virus spread, such as large-scale testing, contact tracing, and isolation of suspected and confirmed cases [49, 50]. Nevertheless, the best preventive measure would be vaccination, but it is impossible to have an effective and safe vaccine available in a short period of time, considering that it is a new virus [51]. The potential vaccines for COVID-19 that are in clinical trials are using different approaches, including live-attenuated virus, viral vectors, inactivated virus, virus-like particles, subunit vaccines, and DNA and RNA vaccines [52]. Regarding therapeutic treatment, there are no drugs currently approved by the US Food and Drug Administration, although several antiviral agents are being tested [53–55]. This situation reinforces the need for alternative measures to prevent the infection while knowledge about the virus is still scarce.

Alternative preventive measures were defined by the WHO in order to reduce the risk of contracting SARS-CoV-2 [56]. One of the recommendations is washing hands regularly with soap and water or using an alcohol-based hand sanitizer to remove the pathogen from the skin [57]. This is possible because soap has a surfactant in its composition that binds with the phospholipid layer of the viral envelope [58, 59]. The act of washing with water helps break the virus's coat, destroying its viability [59]. The antimicrobial activity of the alcohol-based hand sanitizer occurs in an alcohol concentration between 60% and 90% [60]. Alcohol is capable of denaturing proteins by damaging their cytoplasmic membranes, resulting in the release of the genetic material of the virus, capsid destruction, and viral inactivation [61]. In spite of the utmost importance of these hygiene practices, approximately 3 billion people worldwide do not have access to handwashing facilities and 40% of the health facilities lack hand hygiene at points of care [62]. These data reveal the need for better hygiene conditions as a way to maintain the health and quality of life of the population.

To prevent the spread of COVID-19 and other respiratory infections, the WHO also recommends the use of PPE and practice of respiratory hygiene [63]. Face masks, for example, are capable of protecting the wearer from liquid and airborne particles [64]. For this purpose, medical masks or N95 respirators can be used, but the medical mask is effective in preventing larger droplets from reaching the mouth and nose, while the N95 respirator can block out 95% of the smaller (0.3 μ) particles [61]. It is important to highlight that these masks must be worn properly and have to be fit-tested to ensure effectiveness and wearer protection [61, 65]. Considering that hospitals are at risk of running out of masks, the WHO does not recommend that these types of masks be used by people without respiratory symptoms in the community [63]. Currently, it is recommended to wear fabric masks in public settings to reduce transmission from potentially asymptomatic or presymptomatic people [63, 66]. Practicing respiratory hygiene is also recommended, which is the act of covering the mouth and nose with a tissue or with the elbow when coughing or sneezing in order to reduce the transmission through droplets [66]. The preventive measures described here allow people to leave their homes for essential activities, although much has changed in several public and commercial establishments.

Social distancing and quarantine are ways to reduce exposure to SARS-CoV-2 [47]. In community transmission, where links between cases are unclear, social distancing is a useful measure to avoid direct contact with people possibly infected [67]. It involves maintaining a distance of at least 2 m between any two people, prohibiting mass gatherings, limiting the number of people entering stores and supermarkets, and even temporarily closing schools, office buildings, and public spaces [67, 45]. Quarantine was a practice adopted at the start of the COVID-19 outbreak to restrict people who may have been exposed to the virus before it was known they will become ill [68]. In quarantine, home office working is highly encouraged when possible [67]. In cases where home office working is not possible, preventive measures should be adapted to the type of work and the risk of exposure as per the previously cited WHO recommendations [69].

As previously addressed in this chapter, the preventive measures must be strictly followed in health-care facilities because such facilities are at the greatest risk of COVID-19 infection [49]. The concern is not only protecting health-care professionals from illness but also avoiding virus transmission to other patients [65]. For this purpose, it is essential to practice hand hygiene and correctly don and doff PPE [70, 71]. For health-care professionals, the use of masks, gloves, gowns, and goggles is necessary to protect the skin and mucosae from infected body fluids [72]. Rooms should be regularly decontaminated, and the number of visitors have to be limited [67]. In aerosol generating procedures, such as intubation and suction, other airborne precautions should be taken and the equipment must be sterilized before use [71, 65]. Another important issue requiring attention is hospital waste and wastewater, considering that an estimated 25% of the total waste produced by hospitals is hazardous and infectious [73]. Before disposing of, hospital waste and wastewater must be properly treated and disinfected to reduce environmental pollution and the consequent human health risks during the COVID-19 pandemic [55].

Considering the burden on the health-care system, laboratory-confirmed COVID-19 patients with mild disease and no risk factors can be isolated at home [74]. Different from quarantine, isolation is the separation and restriction of ill people to prevent the spread of contagious diseases, like COVID-19 [68]. Even in cases where care is provided at home, many precautions have to be taken and should be adhered to by the patient and household members [74]. A patient must be placed in a well-ventilated single room and personal items that are potentially infectious must not be shared, to avoid virus transmission [71, 74]. Other preventive measures previously mentioned must be taken, such as practicing hand and respiratory hygiene, using PPEs, and maintaining distance from the ill person [65]. In this case, patients and caregivers should use medical masks, while gloves are necessary to handle infectious waste and disinfect surfaces [67, 63]. These wastes, as well as clinical waste, are hazardous to people and have to be identified and collected following strict infection control and hygiene standards [74, 75]. After two negative polymerase chain reaction tests, collected at least 24 hours apart, patients can be released from home isolation [65, 74].

There is still much to understand about SARS-CoV-2, and scientists around the world are sparing no efforts to find answers. Meanwhile, the population should adjust to the new normal with preventive measures and environmental awareness to reduce global spread and avoid future pandemics.

References

1. Chen, N. M. D., Zhou, P. M., Dong, X., Qu, J., Gong, F. and Han, Y. (2020). Epidemiological and clinical characteristics of 99 cases of 2019 novel coronavirus pneumonia in Wuhan, China: a descriptive study, *Lancet*, **395**, pp. 507–513.
2. World Health Organization (2020). Pneumonia of unknown cause – China. Available at <https://www.who.int/csr/don/05-january-2020-pneumonia-of-unkown-cause-china/en/>.
3. National Health Commission of the People's Republic of China (2020). Available at <http://www.nhc.gov.cn/>.

4. Santoso, A. M. D., Pranata, R. M. D., Wibowo, A. M. D., Al-Farabi, M. J., Huang, I. and Antariksa, B. M. D. (2020). Cardiac injury is associated with mortality and critically ill pneumonia in COVID-19: a meta-analysis, *Am. J. Emerg. Med.*, in press.

5. Hui, D. S. C. and Zumla, A. (2019). Severe acute respiratory syndrome: historical, epidemiologic, and clinical features, *Infect. Dis. Clin. North Am.*, **33**, pp. 869–889.

6. Belouzard, S., Millet, J. K., Licitra, B. N. and Whittaker, G. R. (2012). Mechanisms of coronavirus cell entry mediated by the viral spike protein, *Viruses*, **4**, pp. 1011–1033.

7. Hamid, S., Mir, M. Y. and Rohela, G.K. (2020). Novel coronavirus disease (COVID-19): a pandemic (epidemiology, pathogenesis and potential therapeutics), *New Microbes New Infect.*, **35**, p. 100679.

8. Colafrancesco, S., Alessandri, C., Conti, F. and Priori, R. (2020). COVID-19 gone bad: a new character in the spectrum of the hyperferritinemic syndrome?, *Autoimmun. Rev.*, **56**, p. 106053.

9. Bost, P., Giladi, A., Liu, Y., Bendjelal, Y., Xu, G., David, E., Blecher-Gonen, R., Medaglia, C., Li, H., Deczkowska, A., Zhang, S., Schwikowski, B., Zhang, Z. and Amit, I. (2020). Host-viral infection maps reveal signatures of severe COVID-19 patients, *Cell*, pp. 1475–1488.

10. Mahmoud, G., Wang, K., Viveiros, A., Nguyen, Q., Zhong, J., Turner, A. J. and Raizada, M. K. (2020). Angiotensin-converting enzyme 2: SARS-CoV-2 receptor and regulator of the renin-angiotensin system, *Circ. Res.*, **126**, pp. 1456–1474.

11. Joon-Keun, P., Fisher, R., Dechend, R., Shagdarsuren, E., Gapeljuk, A., Wellner, M., Meiners, S., et al. (2007). p38 mitogen-activated protein kinase inhibition ameliorates angiotensin II–induced target organ damage, *Hypertension*, **49**, pp. 481–489.

12. Grimes, J. M. and Grimes, K. V. (2020). p38 MAPK inhibition: a promising therapeutic approach for COVID-19, *JMCC*, **144**, pp. 63–65.

13. Jayaweera, M., Perera, H., Gunawardana, B. and Manatunge, J. (2020). Transmission of COVID-19 virus by droplets and aerosols: a critical review on the unresolved dichotomy, *Environ. Res.*, **188**, p. 109819.

14. Gralton, J., Tovey, E., McLaws, M. and Rawlinson, W. D. (2011). The role of particle size in aerosolised pathogen transmission: a review, *J. Infect.*, **62**, pp. 1–13.

15. Liu, L., Wei, J. and Ooi, A. (2017). Evaporation and dispersion of respiratory droplets from coughing, *Indoor Air*, **27**, pp. 179–190.

16. Hinds, W. C. (1999). *Aerosol Technology: Properties, Behavior, and Measurement of Airborne Particles*, 2nd ed. Wiley, p. 504.

17. World Health Organization (2014). Infection prevention and control of epidemic-and pandemic prone acute respiratory infections in healthcare. WHO guidelines. Available at <http://www.who.int/csr/bioriskreduction/infection_control/publication/en/>.

18. Shiu, E. Y. C., Leung, N. H. L. and Cowling, B. J. (2019). Controversy around airborne versus droplet transmission of respiratory viruses: implication for infection prevention, *Curr. Opin. Infect. Dis.*, **32**, pp. 372–379.

19. Thomas, R. T. (2013). Particle size and pathogenicity in the respiratory tract. *Virulence*, **4**, pp. 847–858.

20. Boone, S. A. and Gerba, C. P. (2007). Significance of fomites in the spread of respiratory and enteric viral disease, *Appl. Environ. Microbiol.*, **73**, pp. 1687–1696.

21. Ong, S. W. X., Tan, Y. K. and Chia, P. Y. (2020). Air, surface environmental, and personal protective equipment contamination by severe acute respiratory syndrome coronavirus 2 (SARS-CoV-2) from a symptomatic patient, *JAMA*, **363**, pp. 1610–1612.

22. Wang, W., Xu, Y. and Gao, R. (2020). Detection of SARS-CoV-2 in different types of clinical specimens, *JAMA*, **323**, pp. 1843–1844.

23. Ahmed, W., Angel, N., Edson, J., Bibby, K., Bivins, A., O'Brien, J. W., et al. (2020). First confirmed detection of SARS-CoV-2 in untreated wastewater in Australia: a proof of concept for the wastewater surveillance of COVID-19 in the community, *Sci. Total Environ.*, **728**, p. 138764.

24. Haramoto, E., Malla, B., Thakali, O. and Kitajima, M. (2020). First environmental surveillance for the presence of SARS-CoV-2 RNA in wastewater and river water in Japan, *Sci. Total Environ.*, **737**, p. 140405.

25. La Rosa, G., Iaconelli, M., Mancini, P., Ferraro, G. B., Veneri, C., Bonadonna, L., et al. (2020). First detection of SARS-CoV-2 in untreated wastewaters in Italy, *Sci. Total Environ.*, **736**, p. 139652.

26. Doremalen, N. V., Bushmaker, T., Morris, D. H., Holdbrook, M. G., Gamble, A., Williamson, B. N., et al. (2020). Aerosol and surface stability of SARS-CoV-2 as compared with SARS-CoV-1, *New Engl. J. Med.*, **382**, pp. 1–4.

27. Tang, J. W., Li, Y., Eames, I., Chan, P. K. S. and Ridgway, G. L. (2006). Factors involved in the aerosol transmission of infection and control of ventilation in healthcare premises, *J. Hosp. Infect.*, **64**, pp. 100–114.

28. Loh, N. Y., Tan, Y., Taculod, J., Gorospe, B., Teope, A. S., Somani, J. and Tan, A. Y. H. (2020). The impact of high-flow nasal cannula (HFNC) on

coughing distance: implications on its use during the novel coronavirus disease outbreak, *Can. J. Anesth.*, **67**, pp. 893–894.

29. Chan, K. H., Peiris, J. S. M., Poon, L. M. M., Yuen, K. Y. and Seto, W. H. (2011). The effects of temperature and relative humidity on the viability of the SARS coronavirus, *Adv. Virol.*, pp. 1–7.

30. Shakil, M. H., Munim, Z. H., Tasnia, M. and Sarowar, S. (2020). COVID-19 and the environment: a critical review and research agenda, *Sci. Total Environ.*, **745**, pp. 141022.

31. Paslakis, G., Dimitropoulos, G. and Katzman, D. K. (2020). A call to action to address COVID-19–induced global food insecurity to prevent hunger, malnutrition, and eating pathology, *Nutr. Rev.*, pp. 1–3.

32. Núñez-Delgado, A. (2020). What do we know about the SARS-CoV-2 coronavirus in the environment?, *Sci. Total Environ.*, **727**, p. 138647.

33. Kumar, M., Patel, A. K., Shah, A. V., Raval, J., Rajpara, N., Joshi, M. and Joshi, C. G. (2020). First proof of the capability of wastewater surveillance for COVID-19 in India through detection of genetic material of SARS-CoV-2, *Sci. Total Environ.*, p. 141326.

34. Heller, L., Mota, C. R. and Greco, D. B. (2020). COVID-19 faecal-oral transmission: are we asking the right questions?, *Sci. Total Environ.*, p. 138919.

35. Kumar, V., Singh, S. B. and Singh, S. (2020). COVID-19: environment concern and impact of indian medicinal system, *J. Environ.*, p. 104144.

36. Saadat, S., Rawtani, D. and Hussain, C. M. (2020). Environmental perspective of COVID-19, *Sci. Total Environ.*, p. 138870.

37. Nguyen, L. H., Drew, D. A., Graham, M. S., Joshi, A. D., Guo, C. G., Ma, W., et al. (2020). Risk of COVID-19 among front-line health-care workers and the general community: a prospective cohort study, *Lancet Public Health*, **5**, E475–E483.

38. Sharma, H. B., Vanapalli, K. R., Cheela, V. S., Ranjan, V. P., Jaglan, A. K., Dubey, B., et al. (2020). Challenges, opportunities, and innovations for effective solid waste management during and post COVID-19 pandemic, *Resour. Conserv. Recy.*, p. 105052.

39. Prata, J. C., Patrício Silva, A. L., Walker, T. R., Duarte, A. C. and Rocha Santos, T. (2020). COVID-19 pandemic repercussions on the use and management of plastics, *Environ. Sci. Technol.*, **54**, pp. 7760–7765.

40. Zambrano-Monserrate, M. A., Ruano, M. A. and Sanchez-Alcalde, L. (2020). Indirect effects of COVID-19 on the environment, *Sci. Total Environ.*, p. 138813.

41. Espejo, W., Celis, J. E., Chiang, G. and Bahamonde, P. (2020). Environment and COVID-19: pollutants, impacts, dissemination, management and recommendations for facing future epidemic threats, *Sci. Total Environ.*, p. 141314.

42. Wang, Q. and Su, M. (2020). A preliminary assessment of the impact of COVID-19 on environment: a case study of China, *Sci. Total Environ.*, p. 138915.

43. Muhammad, S., Long, X. and Salman, M. (2020). COVID-19 pandemic and environmental pollution: a blessing in disguise?, *Sci. Total Environ.*, p. 138820.

44. The European Space Agency (ESA) (2020). Available from: <https://www.esa.int/Applications/Observing_the_Earth/Copernicus/Sentinel-5P>.

45. Chakraborty, I. and Maity, P. (2020). COVID-19 outbreak: migration, effects on society, global environment and prevention, *Sci. Total Environ.*, **728**, p. 138882.

46. Anderson, R. M., Heesterbeek, H., Klinkenberg, D. and Hollingsworth, T. D. (2020). How will country-based mitigation measures influence the course of the COVID-19 epidemic?, *Lancet*, **395**, pp. 21–27.

47. World Health Organization (2020). Responding to community spread of COVID-19. Available at <https://www.who.int/publications/i/item/responding-to-community-spread-of-covid-19>.

48. Ding, Z., Xie, L., Guan, A., Huang, D., Mao, Z. and Liang, X. (2020). Global COVID-19: warnings and suggestions based on experience of China, *J. Glob. Health*, **1**, pp. 1–10.

49. Dhama, K., Khan, S., Tiwari, R., Sircar, S., Bhat, S., Malik, Y. S., Singh, K. P., Chaicumpa, W., Bonilla-Aldana, K. and Rodriguez-Morales, A. J. (2020). Coronavirus disease 2019: COVID-19, *Clin. Microbiol. Rev.*, **33**, pp. 1–48.

50. Singh, V. K., Mishra, A., Singh, S., Kumar, P., Singh, M., Jagannath, C. and Khan, A. (2020). Emerging prevention and treatment strategies to control COVID-19, *Pathogens*, **9**, pp. 2–16.

51. Yang, C., Qiu, X., Fan, H., Jiang, M., Lao, X., Zeng, Y. and Zhang, Z. (2020). Coronavirus disease 2019: reassembly attack of coronavirus, *Int. J. Environ. Health Res.*, **71**, pp. 1–9.

52. Matthew, D. S., Shukla, S., Chung, Y. H., Beiss, V., Chan, S. K., Ortega-Rivera, O. A., Wirth, D. M., Chen, A., Sack, M., Pokorski, J. K. and Steinmetz, N. F. (2020). COVID-19 vaccine development and a potential nanomaterial path forward, *Nat. Nanotechnol.*, **15**, pp. 646–655.

53. Deng, L., Li, C., Zeng, Q., Liu, X., Li, X., Zhang, H., Hong, Z. and Xia, J. (2020). Arbidol combined with LPV/r versus LPV/r alone against Corona Virus Disease 2019: a retrospective cohort study, *J. Infect.*, **81**, pp. e1–e5.

54. Liu, J., Cao, R., Xu, M., Wang, X., Zhang, H., Hu, H., Li, Y., Hu, Z., Zhong, W. and Wang, M. (2020). Hydroxychloroquine, a less toxic derivative of chloroquine, is effective in inhibiting SARS-CoV-2 infection in vitro, *Cell Discov.*, **6**, pp. 1–4.

55. Wang, M., Cao, R., Zhang, L., Yang, X., Liu, J., Xu, M., Shi, Z., Hu, Z., Zhong, W. and Xiao, G. (2020). Remdesivir and chloroquine effectively inhibit the recently emerged novel coronavirus (2019-nCoV) in vitro, *Cell Res.*, **30**, pp. 269–271.

56. World Health Organization (2020). Coronavirus disease (COVID-19) advice for the public. Available at <https://www.who.int/emergencies/diseases/novel-coronavirus-2019/advice-for-public>.

57. Pittet, D., Allegranzi, B., Boyce, J. and WHO (2020). The World Health Organization guidelines on hand hygiene in health care and their consensus recommendations, *Infect. Control Hosp. Epidemiol.*, **30**, pp. 611–622.

58. Ayorinde, F. O., Garvin, K. and Saeed, K. (2000). Determination of the fatty acid composition of saponified vegetable oils using matrix-assisted laser desorption/ionization time-of-flight mass spectrometry, *Rapid Commun. Mass Spectrom.*, **14**, pp. 608–615.

59. Pradhan, D., Biswasroy, P., Naik, P. K., Ghosh, G. and Rath, G. (2020). A review of current interventions for COVID-19 prevention, *Arch. Med. Res.*, **51**, pp. 363–374.

60. McDonnell, G. and Russel, A. D. (1999). Antiseptics and disinfectants: activity, action, and resistance, *Clin. Microbiol. Rev.*, **12**, pp. 147–179.

61. Yan, Y., Shin, W. I., Pang, Y. X., Meng, Y., Lai, J., You, C., Zhao, H., Lester, E., Wu, T. and Pang, C. H. (2020). The first 75 days of novel coronavirus (SARS-CoV-2) outbreak: recent advances, prevention, and treatment, *Int. J. Environ. Res. Public Health*, **17**, pp. 1–23.

62. World Health Organization (2019). Water sanitation hygiene - WASH in health care facilities global baseline report 2019. Available at <https://www.who.int/water_sanitation_health/publications/wash-in-health-care-facilities-global-report/en/>.

63. World Health Organization (2020). Rational use of personal protective equipment for coronavirus disease (COVID-19) and considerations during severe shortages. Available at <https://www.who.int/

publications/i/item/rational-use-of-personal-protective-equipment-for-coronavirus-disease-(covid-19)-and-considerations-during-severe-shortages>.

64. Shiu, E. Y. C., Leung, N. H. L. and Cowling, B. J. (2019). Controversy around airborne versus droplet transmission of respiratory viruses: implication for infection prevention, *Curr. Opin. Infect. Dis.*, **32**, pp. 372–379.

65. Singhal, T. (2020). A review of coronavirus disease-2019 (COVID-19), *Indian J. Pediatr*, **88**, pp. 281–286.

66. Fisher, K. A., Barile, J. P., Guerin, R. J., Esschert, K. L. V., Jeffers, A., Tian, L. H., Gracia-Williams, A., Gurbaxani, B., Thompson, W. W. and Prue, C. R. (2020). Factors associated with cloth face covering use among adults during the COVID-19 pandemic — United States, April and May 2020, *MMWR*, **69**, pp. 933–937.

67. Güner, R., Hassanoglu, I. and Aktas, G. (2020). COVID-19: prevention and control measures in community, *Turk. J. Med. Sci.*, **50**, pp. 571–577.

68. Wilder-Smith, A. and Freedman, D. O. (2020). Isolation, quarantine, social distancing and community containment: pivotal role for old-style public health measures in the novel coronavirus (2019-nCoV) outbreak, *J. Travel Med.*, **2**, pp. 1–4.

69. Occupational Safety and Health Act of 1970 (2020). Guidance on preparing workplaces for COVID-19. Available at <https://www.osha.gov/Publications/OSHA3990.pdf>.

70. Larson, E. L., Early, E., Cloonan, P., Sugrue, S. and Parides, M. (2010). An organizational climate intervention associated with increased handwashing and decreased nosocomial infections, *J. Behav. Med.*, **26**, pp. 14–22.

71. Ouassou, H., Kharchoufa, L., Bouhrim, M., Daoudi, N. E., Imtara, H., Bencheikh, N., Elbouzidi, A. and Bnouham, M. (2020). The pathogenesis of coronavirus disease 2019 (COVID-19): evaluation and prevention, *J. Immunol. Res.*, **20**, pp. 1–7.

72. Meng, L., Hua, F. and Bian, Z. (2020). Coronavirus disease 2019 (COVID-19): emerging and future challenges for dental and oral medicine, *J. Dent. Res.*, **99**, pp. 481–487.

73. World Health Organization (2014). Safe management of wastes from health-care activities. Available at <https://www.who.int/water_sanitation_health/publications/wastemanag/en/>.

74. World Health Organization (2020). Home care for patients with suspected or confirmed COVID-19 and management of their contacts.

Available at <https://www.who.int/publications/i/item/home-care-for-patients-with-suspected-novel-coronavirus-(ncov)-infection-presenting-with-mild-symptoms-and-management-of-contacts>.

75. Nghiem, L. D., Morgan, B., Donner, E. and Short, M. (2020). The COVID-19 pandemic: considerations for the waste and wastewater services sector, *CSCEE*, **1**, p. 100006.

Chapter 2

Environmental Fate of COVID-19

Daniela Montanari Migliavacca Osório, Alessa Maria Ceratti, Darlan Daniel Alves, Eduarda Sthefanie Mittelstadt, Fernando Luzardo Rabelo, Filipe Brochier, Júlia Luz Bohrer, Vanusca Dalosto Jahno, and Daniela Müller de Quevedo

Feevale University, ERS-239, 2755, 93525-075, Novo Hamburgo, Rio Grande do Sul, Brazil
danielaosorio@feevale.br

At the end of 2019, the world faced a new virus, SARS-CoV-2, which is currently present in almost every country in the world. In this sense, the World Health Organization (WHO) has classified the pandemic as a high global risk, which made important the actions to understand and elucidate the behavior of this new virus, as well as its consequences for humanity. We are still trying to understand how it propagates in the environment, whether through air, via object surfaces, or even by wastewaters and natural waters. In atmospheric air, studies indicate an association between the air quality index (AQI) and the confirmed cases of COVID-19 in several cities in China, as well as an association between the transmission of COVID-19 by air and meteorological variables, suggesting that temperature conditions in the range of 10°C–20°C and humidity between 10% and 20% may present risks. In contrast, some studies indicate an improvement in the air quality due to a reduction in

Living with COVID-19: Economics, Ethics, and Environmental Issues
Edited by Chaudhery Mustansar Hussain and Gustavo Marques da Costa
Copyright © 2022 Jenny Stanford Publishing Pte. Ltd.
ISBN 978-981-4877-78-7 (Hardcover), 978-1-003-16828-7 (eBook)
www.jennystanford.com

vehicle and industrial emissions, enforcement of social distance, and even lockdown. Analyses of wastewaters from domestic sewage have revealed the presence of viral genetic material in the feces and urine of infected individuals, which proves the presence of the virus in this matrix. It was also noticed that SARS-CoV-2-like viruses persist in natural waters and sewers for more than 10 days. The transmission of the virus via the fecal-oral route due to contact with contaminated sewage water has not yet been proven and, therefore, this possibility cannot be ruled out. Also, a deep reflection on the establishment of protocols for the management of solid health residues with eminent contamination by COVID-19 is necessary. Given the questions and doubts regarding the behavior of this new virus in the environment, this chapter will compile studies related to the transport of COVID-19 in the environment, in order to assist in the development of preventive and protective measures against this new virus.

2.1 COVID-19 Lifetime on Surfaces

According to recent research, Coronavirus Disease 2019 (COVID-19) can remain on different surfaces of materials for up to 9 days [8, 22]. Transmission among the population occurs both in hospital and family settings, and it is important to avoid any spread in the public and in health-care facilities. The transmission of COVID-19 on contaminated surfaces has been studied more because it facilitates self-infection through the mucous membranes of the eyes, mouth, and nose [17, 31].

Previous studies have shown that the severe acute respiratory syndrome (SARS) coronavirus and other coronaviruses can survive on environmental surfaces and inanimate objects. However, the new 2019 coronavirus has not been reported in the environment. According to the WHO, there is no certainty about how long the COVID-19 virus survives on surfaces, but it appears to act like other coronaviruses. Preliminary studies show that coronaviruses, including the COVID-19 virus, can remain on surfaces from several hours to several days. This can vary under different circumstances (e.g., type of surface, ambient temperature, and humidity).

A study published by Suman et al. [43] on the sustainability of the coronavirus on different surfaces indicated that the viral load of SARS-CoV-2 was higher in plastics and stainless steel, at 72 hours and 48 hours, respectively, and in aerosol, it can remain viable for 3 hours. However, on copper and cardboard surfaces, viral viability was not identified in 4 and 24 hours, respectively. The same behavior of SARS-CoV-2 was observed in the experiment proposed by van Doremalen [16], where the virus remained viable in aerosols for 3 hours, with a reduction in viral load from 103.5 to 102.7 TCID50 per liter of air, showing the same behavior with other materials, plastic, stainless steel, copper, and cardboard. SARS-CoV-2 is also more stable on smooth surfaces [10]. Table 2.1 shows the persistence of coronavirus on different surfaces.

SARS-CoV-2 can be highly stable in a favorable environment, that is, environmental conditions can favor its permanence for a longer time, which is a common characteristic of enveloped viruses, such as human coronaviruses. Environmental parameters such as heat, humidity, pH, and type of surface influence the viability of these viruses, and environmental surfaces are likely to contribute to the spread of viral infections derived from hospitals [21, 34].

Table 2.1 Coronavirus persistence on different surfaces

Surface	Maximum viability time
Aerosol	3 hours (half-life 1.2 hours)
Plastic	Up to 72 hours (half-life of 6.8 hours) in a study comparing SARS-CoV-1 and SARS-CoV-2 /up to 9 days under review with other coronaviruses
Stainless steel	Up to 72 hours (half-life 5.6 hours)
Copper	4 hours
Cardboard	24 hours
Aluminum	2–8 hours
Metal	5 days
Wood	4 days
Paper	5 days
Glass	5 days
Glove (latex)	8 hours
Disposable apron	2 days
Ceramics	5 days

Source: Adapted from Refs. [16, 22].

The survival time of the virus that causes COVID-19 on surfaces is not yet adequately known, but it apparently resembles that of other coronaviruses. Recently, a review of the viability of human coronaviruses on surfaces revealed a high survival capacity, in the range of 2 hours to 9 days [46]. Encapsulated viruses showed more sensitivity than nonencapsulated viruses when the liquid-air interface was lower (when there was less relative humidity in the environments) [21] and can also survive for days or even weeks on dry, hydrophobic surfaces [18, 45]. Coronaviruses are encapsulated and usually have greater vulnerability to acidic pH, basic pH, and heat, and their casing is sensitive to dryness, which, in this case, facilitates their sterilization process [18, 45].

Surface contamination in hospitals was investigated by Razzini et al. [33]. They reported that 35% of the surfaces in the COVID-19 patients' ward were contaminated with COVID-19, 50% of the surfaces in the undressing room were contaminated with the same, and there was no COVID-19 contamination of surfaces in the clean area. The most contaminated surfaces were dispensers of hand disinfectants, medical equipment, touch screens of medical equipment, shelves for medical equipment, grids, and handles. Virus inactivation can be achieved after 1 min. with the use of surface disinfectants such as ethanol (62%–71%), hydrogen peroxide (0.5%), or sodium hypochlorite (0·1%), but other biocides, such as benzalkonium chloride (0 $\pm$ 0.5% to 0 $\pm$ 2%) or chlorhexidine digluconate (0 $\pm$ 0.2%) were less effective [22].

2.2 Presence of COVID-19 in Atmospheric Air/Decline in Air Pollution due to COVID-19 Lockdown

2.2.1 Presence of COVID-19 in Atmospheric Air

Since the WHO public health emergency declaration of international interest issued on the SARS-CoV-2 virus on January 30, 2020, when there were still less than 100 cases and no deaths outside China, studies have been evaluating the association between confirmed cases and mortality by COVID-19 and the concentration of air pollutants, such as particulate matter (PM), nitrogen dioxide (NO_2), nitrogen monoxide (NO), sulfur dioxide (SO_2), carbon monoxide (CO), and ozone (O_3) [3, 12, 26, 35, 37]; meteorological factors [1, 24, 25, 37, 54, 55]; and decrease in atmospheric pollution due to lockdown [9, 24, 26, 30, 37, 39].

Air pollution has been shown to be responsible for killing about 7 million people a year [47]. As if that were not enough, studies have been showing that exposure to high levels of air pollutants in the short and long term contributes to an increase in the cases of COVID-19 [12, 54].

However, in order to contain the increase in COVID-19 cases, many countries have adopted the lockdown method, with the aim of keeping the population in social isolation [2, 26], which, consequently, has been improving local AQIs [2, 30, 37].

Almost a third of Chinese cities joined the lockdown, improving local air quality, which made it possible to verify that the effects of the blockade were greater in colder, richer, and more industrialized cities. Consequently, due to the reduction in atmospheric pollution, an evident health benefit was perceived. However, the economic interruption caused by a lockdown can negatively impact health in the long term [19].

According to the Center for Research on Energy and Clean Air, social isolation and the drop in industrial and vehicular activities in Europe resulted in a reduction of approximately 40% in the NO_2 levels and 10% in the PM levels in just 30 days; as a result, there were 11,000 fewer deaths by air pollution. In addition to the drop of 1.3 million days of absenteeism at work, there were 6000 fewer new cases of asthma among children, 1900 fewer visits to emergencies due to asthma exacerbation, and 600 fewer premature births due to chronic exposure to air pollutants [7].

However, lockdown is an inefficient measure to achieve pollution reduction; there are numerous other, cheaper strategies to achieve this environmental goal [19]. It should be noted that the COVID-19 crisis has had immeasurable impacts on the population worldwide, and these data indicate that not only the air quality but also the quality of life for all of humanity can improve rapidly as the main pollution sources are eliminated. This is just a demonstration of how public health can be improved once sustainable measures are adopted [7]. However, for scientists, researchers, students, and individuals in general, it is an opportunity to understand through the application of the lockdown the interaction and the behavior of the levels of atmospheric pollutants in the face of an economic slowdown, aiming to find an alternative for the long term [44].

Researchers realized that airborne transmission of the COVID-19 virus is a real risk [29] and that exposure to air pollution, coupled with specific weather conditions, is probably contributing to the spread of the virus [7, 13, 55], especially among populations living in areas with high levels of pollutants, as they are already living in an environment that induces a chronic inflammatory process, which makes them more susceptible to respiratory and cardiovascular diseases [12].

At the epicenter of the disease in Italy, in the city of Bergamo, research showed the presence of SARS-CoV-2 RNA in PM_{10}. This was the first research to find the virus RNA in PM, suggesting its possible use as a recurrence indicator epidemic, especially as high levels of pollution decrease the natural defenses of the human body, making it more likely to contract viral diseases, such as Sars-Cov-2 [36].

In Italy, the population of the north of the country was also studied for the risk of exposure to air pollutants. Also studied were the effects of short-term exposure to PM_{10} and NO_2 in Lombardy, where increased concentrations of pollutants were associated with increased mortality and hospital admissions. According to the study, it can be assumed that prolonged cellular oxidative stress, induced by inhaled pollutants, can predispose a person's respiratory system to a severe impact of viruses. In this context, it is possible that some pollutants, specifically $PM_{2.5}$ and PM_{10}, may favor not only the pathogenicity of the virus but also its spread. Bearing in mind that they are inhalable particles, they constitute a health risk, increasing the risk of mortality from infections and respiratory diseases [35, 49, 50]. As the virus survives for a few hours and even days, it can be assumed that specific atmospheric conditions can facilitate its spread [35].

2.2.2 Decline in Air Pollution due to COVID-19 Lockdown

Several countries have taken measures to mitigate the transmission of SARS-CoV-2 in order to stem the spread of the disease. These measures have generated economic and social impacts, reflecting in the drop in industrial activities and vehicular traffic, positively impacting air quality in several regions in the world [4, 11, 30, 44].

It was possible to verify that air quality can improve quickly as soon as pollution sources are suppressed [14, 44], as observed in countries like China [44], India [26], Italy [11], Malaysia [23], and Brazil [14, 30].

A reduction can be seen in the main air pollutants, including $PM_{2.5}$, PM_{10}, CO, SO_2, NO_2, NH_3, NO_x, and benzene. In contrast, an increase can be seen in O_3 [11, 14, 24, 26, 30, 37, 44], which may be due to the decrease in the levels of PM and NO_x [37], since NO is responsible for the titration of tropospheric O_3 [38]. However, climatic conditions influence the concentration of pollutants present in the atmosphere [37]. Meteorological factors play an independent role in the transmission of COVID-19, favoring transmission in a climate with low temperature, light daytime temperature range, and low humidity [25, 54]. Meteorological indicators are significant and essential in the forecast and prevention of the transmission of COVID-19 [55].

It should be noted that although the lockdown may have contributed to the improvement in the world's air quality, one must take into account the social and economic negative impacts that the pandemic has brought to society [30].

The air pollution in the megacity of Delhi, India, after 3 weeks of lockdown, showed a considerable decrease in its levels, with decreasing trends in the concentrations of PM_{10}, $PM_{2.5}$, NO_2, and CO; there was a decrease of 51.84% and 53.11% in the concentrations of PM_{10} and $PM_{2.5}$, respectively, in relation to the months before the lockdown. However, when compared to the same period of previous years, the concentrations indicated a variation of −56.55% and −32.62% in the concentrations of PM_{10} and $PM_{2.5}$, respectively [26].

In the United States, a study was carried out in approximately 3000 municipalities, covering over 85% of the population, where the relationship between exposure to air pollutants and COVID-19 mortality was analyzed. It was concluded that an increase of only 1 $\mu g/m^3$ in $PM_{2.5}$ levels is associated with a 15% increase in the mortality rate due to COVID-19 [51].

The effect of the lockdown on air quality was assessed in four southern European cities (Nice, Rome, Valencia, and Turin) and in the Chinese city of Wuhan, focusing on the concentrations of O_3. Compared to the same period from 2017 to 2019, the average daily O_3 concentrations increased in urban stations by 24% in Nice, 14% in Rome, 27% in Turin, 2.4% in Valencia, and 36% in Wuhan during the lockdown of 2020. The increase in O_3 occurred mainly due to a large decrease in NO emissions, largely from the transport sector. On the other hand, during the lockdown, domestic activities that emit precursors of O_3 increased, such as CO and volatile organic compounds. Also due to lower concentrations of PM_{10} and $PM_{2.5}$, an increase in solar radiation favored the formation of O_3 [38].

In the United States, the State of California has the worst air quality according to recent studies. Of the country's 25 most polluted cities, 10 are in California. The establishment of the mandatory lockdown resulted in a reduction in environmental pollutants by up to 60%. Data were collected from March 4 to April 24, 2020, to assess air pollutants. Significant correlations were found between PM_{10}, $PM_{2.5}$, SO_2, CO, and NO_2 and the total cases and total deaths in the state in both Spearman and Kendall correlations. However, the magnitudes of the correlation coefficients for PM_{10}, $PM_{2.5}$, SO_2, Pb, and NO_2 were higher in the Spearman correlation test. The study suggests that the adoption of environmental laws should be promoted as a measure to protect human life, especially the lives of children and older adults, who are the most vulnerable to infectious diseases [3].

As a probable side effect of the 69.85% reduction in mobility, production, and consumption activities, many regions recorded a decrease in air pollution, strongly associated with mobility restrictions during the pandemic. On average, the AQI decreased by 7.8% and the levels of the pollutants SO_2, $PM_{2.5}$, PM_{10}, NO_2, and CO decreased by 6.76%, 5.93%, 13.66%, 24.67%, and 4.58%, respectively. PM_{10} and NO_2 showed the biggest reductions. This is due to the fact that these pollutants result primarily from the vehicular exhaust and road dust generated in transportation activities. For the AQI, $PM_{2.5}$, and CO, the relationship was partially mediating between the movement of people and the reduction in pollutants. As for SO_2, PM_{10}, and NO_2, the relationship was totally mediating, that is, 100% of the pollutant variation was due to the reduction in population mobility [2].

In Malaysia, researchers have studied the effects of lockdown on air quality due to the reduction in $PM_{2.5}$ levels recorded by all 68 monitoring stations in the country. Before and during the implementation of the lockdown, $PM_{2.5}$ concentrations ranged from 5.3 to 42.5 $\mu g/m^3$ and from 3.9 to 69.2 $\mu g/m^3$, respectively. The reductions occurred in a total of 34 monitoring stations—50% of the stations. The station with the highest level of reduction (Politeknik Kota Kinabalu) recorded a 58.5% decrease in $PM_{2.5}$ concentrations. In Malaysia, the lockdown was divided into two phases, included in the study, and a third phase was implemented after the studies was carried out [1].

Chauhan and Singh [9] assessed the pollutant $PM_{2.5}$ and the atmospheric precipitation in the period of December 2019 to March 2020 and compared these with periods of previous years (2017 to 2019) for the cities of New York, Los Angeles, Zaragoza, Rome, Dubai, Delhi, Mumbai, Beijing, and Shanghai, which were in a lockdown mode in March 2020. In New York, for the month of March 2020, there was a 32% reduction in the $PM_{2.5}$ level compared to the level in March 2019 and a 20% reduction compared to that in February 2020. In Los Angeles, there was a reduction of 4% in the $PM_{2.5}$ level when compared to the levels in March 2020 and March 2019 and a 30% reduction compared to that in February 2020, and in this case, the influence of precipitation on the results was verified. In Zaragoza, Spain, there was a 58% reduction in $PM_{2.5}$ levels compared to the levels in March 2020 and 2019. In Rome, Italy, in March 2020, the $PM_{2.5}$ level was 24% lower when compared to the level in March 2019. In Dubai, the reduction in the $PM_{2.5}$ level in the same months was 11%. In India, in the cities of Delhi and Mumbai, a reduction of 35% and 14%, respectively, was observed. Finally, in the Chinese cities of Beijing and Shanghai, reductions of 50% in $PM_{2.5}$ levels were observed in the month of March 2020 in comparison to the level in the same month in 2019.

Through the studies presented, the importance of public policies aligned with the reduction of air pollutants is verified, given the indisputable association between the AQI and public health and, as evidenced by the pandemic COVID-19, between the AQI and anthropogenic activities [2, 6, 38, 44].

2.3 Studies of COVID-19 in Sewage Water

COVID-19 is an infectious disease whose causative agent is the SARS-CoV-2 virus. Its main symptoms are fever, cough or sore throat, and/or difficulty in breathing. However, in some cases, the disease can cause gastrointestinal symptoms, like diarrhea.

The transmission of COVID-19 can occur through two main routes: the airway and contact with contaminated aerosols. However, recent research suggests a third route of transmission, the fecal-oral, where the individual comes in contact with wastewater. As it is a very complex mechanism of transmission, this is a possibility, but it is not conclusive [5]. In recent months, due to the virus's high dissemination around the world, studies have revealed the presence of fragments of the viral genetic material in the excretions of infected individuals and, consequently, in sewage waters [42]. Contaminated wastewaters increase the circulation of the virus, in addition to increasing the viral load in the local sewage system [28]. The persistence of SARS-CoV-2-like viruses in natural waters and sewers was observed for more than 10 days. In low-income countries, hospital wastewaters are directly discharged untreated into sewage systems, and this can introduce infectious agents such as SARS-CoV-2 into the environment, which can cause both environmental and public health problems [27].

Consideration should be given to the limited access of the general population to safe drinking water, as well as the lack of basic sanitation in various locations around the world. In Brazil, despite the existence of a National Basic Sanitation Plan, only about 60.9% of Brazilian cities have sewage collection networks. On top of that, the country's sewage treatment takes care of only 46.3% of the estimated wastewaters generated and 74.5% of the sewage collected [40]. Estimates worldwide indicate that about 1.8 billion people consume water contaminated with feces, 2.2 billion individuals do not have access to safe drinking water, and 4.2 billion individuals are deprived of safely managed sanitation [20].

Due to the high transmissibility of COVID-19 and the overburdened health services worldwide, the current scenario requires urgent measures to reduce the progression of the virus, which can be taken through early diagnosis and social isolation. A tool that is being used is sewage surveillance, which has been shown to be a good indicator for monitoring the spread of viruses in the population, making it possible to notify new outbreaks of the disease, as well as indicating control of the global pandemic, even before confirmation of positive cases of COVID-19, serving as an early warning of new cases. Sewage monitoring actions can assist in the surveillance and monitoring of the virus circulation among the population, making it possible to take control measures in a timely manner [42].

A strategy that has already been used for tracking and signaling outbreaks of viral diseases is wastewater-based epidemiology (WBE). It is effective in detecting viral particles, as it uses the reverse transcription-quantitative polymerase chain reaction, commonly known as RT-qPCR, which makes it possible to identify and quantify RNA in samples [41].

Although there are no absolute data on the viable SARS-CoV-2 load and its transmissibility through the water used for recreational activities, bathing, and drinking, the best strategy to stop its spread via the fecal-oral route is to treat the water before ingestion [5]. But the lack of treatment of cloacal sewage in some parts of the world can enhance this transmission route, which can lead to a considerable risk of contamination.

Researchers found a high viral titer of SARS-CoV-2 in the wastewater at an urban treatment plant in Massachusetts, US, in March 2020 [51]. In the Netherlands, it was possible to observe a correlation between the increase in viral RNA fragments in wastewater and the increased prevalence of the disease in the country [28]. In Amersfoort, Netherlands, virus fragments were detected in the sewer 6 days before the first cases were reported, which indicates that sewage can be a sensitive tool for monitoring the virus in the population [28].

WBE can be a very efficient strategy for the identification of SARS-CoV-2 in places where testing for COVID-19 is still incipient or even insignificant. The process of transmission of COVID-19 through the oral-fecal route still requires further studies. The presence of SARS-CoV-2 in the feces of infected patients indicates that it is necessary to be alert, since insects such as flies and cockroaches can become important transmitters of COVID-19 once they have the potential to transmit other pathogens, such as bacteria and parasites, in addition to other viruses [15].

It should be noted that even if investigations indicate the presence of SARS-CoV-2 in the feces of infected people, the detection of viral RNA alone does not indicate the presence of the live virus, but it is a warning, and researchers from all over the world are investigating this type transmission route, with some finding positive results for the presence of SARS-CoV-2 in human feces [53].

Wastewater is an important tool for future studies aimed at prevention, early detection, and pandemic management and can help improve the response in terms of safety measures and containment of the disease [27]. The pandemic is considered a complex situation, being aggravated by the lack of economic resources and degradation of environmental conditions, especially in low-income countries, signaling the need for studies that enable the development of new schemes and methodologies to combat SARS-CoV-2 [27].

2.4 Protocols for Managing Health-Care Waste with COVID-19

Health-care waste carries several pathogenic agents, and this leads to the risk of contamination, both directly and indirectly, if the protocols for handling and treatment of this waste are not strictly followed. Appropriate personal protective equipment (PPE), such as masks, gloves, long-sleeved aprons, goggles, and whatever else is needed for the generation site and indicated by the work environment safety plans, is required for handling this waste [21].

With the worldwide establishment of the COVID-19 pandemic, all actions to contain the virus have produced a huge amount of solid health waste. The composition of this waste is usually disposable plastic, often from PPE, drug vials and packaging, and related products. This is causing an environmental and public health crisis around the world, especially in countries where there are no public policies for the management and management of solid health-care waste [39].

New studies since the beginning of the pandemic indicate that PPE can be disinfected by methods such as ultraviolet irradiation, application of spray disinfectants, and application of various types of infusion (whether with nanotechnology or hydrogen peroxide), enabling the reuse of the PPE. These disinfection methods are in the preliminary study phase or have to be applied on a large scale, which is not economically feasible for many countries. In addition, it is important to ensure that after being disinfected, the PPE still maintains its pathogen protection function [32].

The WHO has released guidelines for the disposal of contaminated and uncontaminated waste during the COVID-19 outbreak, and the proportion of uncontaminated waste is greater than 80% of the total amount of health-care waste generated, which needs to be collected and disposed of in landfills [47].

The standards of good practice in the management of health-care waste should be followed, ensuring safe segregation and disposal of the waste. Whether transmission occurs during handling of health-care waste is still under study, and infectious waste (infectious, sharp, and pathological waste) should be safely collected in lined containers or double plastic bags and clearly identified. This waste should be treated, preferably on-site, and then safely disposed of. Everyone dealing with health-care waste should wear PPE (boots, long-sleeved gown, heavy duty gloves, mask, and goggles or a face shield) and perform hand hygiene after removing it. It is preferable to treat these wastes using technological treatment alternatives, such as autoclave and incinerators.

The COVID-19 pandemic has posed a challenge in the area of health waste, which will continue to be generated in large quantities, requiring each country to invest in studies to reduce this contaminated waste and improve its management.

2.5 Conclusion

According to the various studies covered in this chapter, it was possible to identify the presence of SARS-CoV-2 in the air and in wastewater. Although no study has indicated the spread of the virus through contact with contaminated water or through air pollution particles, the relevance of expanding studies in these areas is evident, such as the identification of its infection potential when evidenced in these environments. This is a new virus, and science is still looking for more accurate information about its spread, effective security measures, and even the possibility of reinfection and mutations that have already occurred in the virus.

Studies capable of modeling the behavior of the spread of the virus in conjunction with social and environmental vulnerabilities will also be of great importance in the establishment of specific and efficient actions for the containment of the disease and, mainly, for the protection of individuals from risk groups. It is expected that positive results in relation to the various vaccines being tested at the moment will be obtained as soon as possible. However, there is still a long way to go before the production of an effective vaccine on a large scale and that can be made available to the vast majority of the population. Thus, it is expected that actions arising from scientific research and that expand knowledge about SARS-CoV-2 in terms of propagation in various media and systems and that result in efficient protection protocols will emerge.

References

1. Abdullah, S., Mansor, A. A., Napi, N. N. L. M., Mansor, W. N. W., Ahmed, A. N., Ismail, M. and Ramly, Z. T. A. (2020). Air quality status during 2020 Malaysia Movement Control Order (MCO) due to 2019 novel coronavirus (2019-nCoV) pandemic, *Sci. Total Environ.*, **729**, p. 139022. https://doi.org/10.1016/j.scitotenv.2020.139022.

2. Bao, R. and Zhang, A. (2020). Does lockdown reduce air pollution? Evidence from 44 cities in northern China, *Sci. Total Environ*, **731**, p. 139052. https://doi.org/10.1016/j.scitotenv.2020.139052.

3. Bashir, M. F., Bilal, B. M. and Komal, B. (2020). Correlation between environmental pollution indicators and COVID-19 pandemic: a brief study in Californian context, *Environ. Res.*, **187**, p. 109652. https://doi.org/10.1016/j.envres.2020.109652.

4. Berman, J. B. and Ebisu, K. (2020). Changes in U.S air pollution during the COVID-19 pandemic, *Sci. Total Environ.*, **739**, p. 139864. https://doi.org/10.1016/j.scitotenv.2020.139864.

5. Bhowmick, G. D., Dhar, D., Nath, D., Makarand, G. M., Banerjee, R., Das, S. and Chatterjee, J. (2020). Coronavirus disease 2019 (COVID-19) outbreak: some serious consequences with urban and rural water cycle, *NPJ Clean Water*, **3**, pp. 1–8. https://doi.org/10.1038/s41545-020-0079-1.

6. Bontempi, E. (2020). First data analysis about possible COVID-19 virus airborne diffusion due to air particulate matter (PM): the case of Lombardy (Italy), *Environ. Res.*, **186** p. 109639. https://doi.org/10.1016/j.envres.2020.109639.

7. Centre for Research on Energy and Clean Air (CREA) (2020). 11,000 air pollution-related deaths avoided in Europe as coal, oil consumption plummet. https://energyandcleanair.org/air-pollution-deaths-avoided-in-europe-as-coal-oil-plummet.

8. Chan, J. F, Yuan, S., Kok, K. H, To, K. K., Chu, H. and Yang, J. (2020). A familial cluster of pneumonia associated with the 2019 novel coronavirus indicating person-to-person transmission: a study of a family cluster, *Lancet*, **395**, pp. 514–523. https://doi.org/10.1016/S0140-6736(20)30154-9.

9. Chauhan, A. and Singh, R. P. (2020). Decline in PM2.5 concentrations over major cities around the world associated with COVID-19, *Environ. Res.*, **187**, p. 109634. https://doi.org/10.1016/j.envres.2020.109634.

10. Chin, A. W. H., Chu, J. T. S., Perera, M. R. A., Hui, K. P. Y., Yen, H. L., Chan, M. C. W., Peiris, M. and Poon, L. L. M. (2020). Stability of SARS-CoV-2 in different environmental conditions. *Lancet*, **1**, p. 1. https://doi.org/10.1016/S2666-5247(20)30003-3.

11. Collivignarelli, M. C., Abbà, A., Bertanza, G., Pedrazzani, R., Ricciardi, P. and Carnevale Miino, M. (2020). Lockdown for CoViD-2019 in Milan: what are the effects on air quality?, *Sci. Total. Environ.*, **732**, p. 139280. https://doi.org/10.1016/j.scitotenv.2020.139280.

12. Comunian, S., Dongo, D., Milani, C. and Palestini, P. (2020). Air pollution and COVID-19: the role of particulate matter in the spread and increase of COVID-19's morbidity and mortality. *Int. J. Environ. Res. Public Health*, **17**, pp. 1–22. https://doi.org/10.3390/ijerph17124487.

13. Conticini, E., Frediani, B. and Caro, D. (2020). Can atmospheric pollution be considered a co-factor in extremely high level of SARS-CoV-2 lethality in Northern Italy?, *Environ. Pollut.*, **261**, p. 114465. https://doi.org/10.1016/j.envpol.2020.114465.

14. Dantas, G., Siciliano, B., França, B., Silva, C. and Arbilla, G. (2020). The impact of COVID-19 partial lockdown on the air quality of the city of Rio de Janeiro, Bazil, *Sci. Total Environ.*, **729**, p. 139085. https://doi.org/10.1016/j.scitotenv.2020.139085.

15. Dehghani, R. and Kassiri, H. (2020). A brief review on the possible role of houseflies and cockroaches in the mechanical transmission of coronavirus disease 2019 (COVID-2010), *Arch. Clin. Infect. Dis.*, Online ahead of print., **15**(COVID-19), p. e102863. doi:10.5812/archcid.102863.

16. Van Doremalen, N., Morris, D. H., Holbrook, M. G., Gamble, A., Williamson, B., Tamin, A., Lloyd-Smith, J. and Wit, E., (2020). Aerosol and surface stability of SARS-CoV-2 as compared with SARS-CoV-1, *N. Engl. J. Med.*, **16**, p. 382. doi:10.1056/NEJMc2004973.

17. Dowell, S. F, Simmerman, J. M., Erdman, D. D., Wu, J. S., Chaovavanich, A. and Javadi, M. (2004). Severe acute respiratory syndrome coronavirus on hospital surfaces, *Clin. Infect. Dis.*, **39**, pp. 652–657.

18. Firquet, S., Beaujard, S., Lobert, P., Sané, F., Caloone, D., Izard, D. and Hober, D. (2015). Survival of enveloped and non-enveloped viruses on inanimate surfaces, *Microbes Environ.*, **30**, pp. 140–144. doi:10.1264/jsme2.ME14145.

19. He, G., Pan, Y. and Tanaka, T. (2020). The short-term impacts of COVID-19 lockdown on urban air pollution in China, *Nat. Sustain.*, https://doi.org/10.1038/s41893-020-0581-y.

20. Heller, L., Mota, C. R. and Greco, D. B. (2020). COVID-19 faecal-oral transmission: are we asking the right questions?, *Sci. Total Environ.*, **729**, p. 138919. https://doi.org/10.1016/j.scitotenv.2020.138919.

21. Hoseinzadeh, E., Safoura, J., Farzadkia, M., Mohammadi, F., Hossini, H. and Taghavi, M. (2020). An updated min-review on environmental route of the SARS-CoV-2 transmission, *Ecotoxicol. Environ. Saf.*, **202**, p. 111015. doi:10.1016/j.ecoenv.2020.111015.

22. Kampf, G., Todt, D., Pfaender, S. and Steinmann, E., (2020). Persistence of coronaviruses on inanimate surfaces and their inactivation with biocidal agents, *J. Hosp. Infect.*, **104**, pp. 246–251. doi:10.1016/j.jhin.2020.01.022.

23. Kanniah, K. D., Zaman, N. A. F. K., Kaskaoutis, D. G. and Latif, M. T. (2020). COVID-19's impact on the atmospheric environment

in the Southeast Asia region, *Sci. Total Environ.*, **736**, p. 139658. doi:10.1016/j.scitotenv.2020.139658.

24. Kerimray, A., Baimatova, N., Ibragimova, O. P., Bukenov, B., Kenessov, B., Plotitsyn, P. and Karaca, F. (2020). Assessing air quality changes in large cities during COVID-19 lockdowns: the impacts of traffic-free urban conditions in Almaty, Kazakhstan, *Sci. Total Environ.*, **730**, p. 139179. https://doi.org/10.1016/j.scitotenv.2020.139179.

25. Liu, J., Zhou, J., Yao, J., Zhang, X., Li, L., Xu, X. and Zhang, K. (2020). Impact of meteorological factors on the COVID-19 transmission: a multi-city study in China, *Sci. Total Environ.*, **726**, p. 138513. https://doi.org/10.1016/j.scitotenv.2020.138513.

26. Mahato, S., Pal, S. and Ghosh, K. G. (2020). Effect of lockdown amid COVID-19 pandemic on air quality of the megacity Delhi, India, *Sci. Total Environ.*, **730**, p. 139086. https://doi.org/10.1016/j.scitotenv.2020.139086.

27. Mandi, L. (2020). Urgent needs to consider and assess the transmission of coronavirus (COVID-19) via hospital sewage and wastewater, *J. Clin. Exp. Invest.*, **11**, pp. 1–3. https://doi.org/10.5799/jcei/8261.

28. Medema, G., Heijnen, L., Elsinga, G., Italiaander, R. and Brouwer, A. (2020). Presence of SARS-coronavirus-2 RNA in sewage and correlation with reported COVID-19 prevalence in the early stage of the epidemic in the Netherlands environ, *Sci. Technol. Lett.*, **7**, pp. 511–516. https://doi.org/10.1021/acs.estlett.0c00357.

29. Morawska, L. and Milton, D. K. (2020). It is time to address airborne transmission of COVID-19, *Clin. Infect. Dis.*, **ciaa939**, pp. 1–9. https://doi.org/10.1093/cid/ciaa939.

30. Nakada, L. Y. K. and Urban, R. C. (2020). COVID-19 pandemic: impacts on the air quality during the partial lockdown in São Paulo state, Brazil, *Sci. Total Environ.*, **730**, p. 139087. https://doi.org/10.1016/j.scitotenv.2020.139087.

31. Otter, J. A., Donskey, C., Yezli, S., Douthwaite, S., Goldenberg, S. D. and Weber, D. J. (2016). Transmission of SARS and MERS coronaviruses and influenza virus in healthcare settings: the possible role of dry surface contamination, *J. Hosp. Infect.*, **92**, pp. 235–250. doi:10.1016/j.jhin.2015.08.027.

32. Price, A. D., Cui, Y., Liao, L., Xiao, W., Yu, X., Wang, H., Zhao, M., Wang, Q., Chu, S. and Chu, L. F. (2020). Is the fit of N95 facial masks effected by disinfection? A study of heat and UV disinfection methods using the OSHA protocol fit test, *medRxiv*, pp. 1–21. https://doi.org/10.1101/2020.04.14.20062810.

33. Razzini, K., Castrica, M., Menchetti, L., Maggi, L., Negroni, L. Orfeo, N., V., Pizzoccheri, A., Stocco, M., Muttini, S. and Balzaretti, C. (2020). SARS-CoV-2 RNA detection in the air and on surfaces in the COVID-19 ward of a hospital in Milan, Italy. *Sci Total Environ.*, **742**, p. 140540. https://doi.org/10.1016/j.scitotenv.2020.140540.

34. Ryu, B., Cho, Y., Cho, O., Hong, S., Kim, S. and Lee, S. (2020). Environmental contamination of SARS-CoV-2 during the COVID-19 outbreak in South Korea, *Am. J. Infect. Control*, **48**, pp. 875–879. https://doi.org/10.1016/j.ajic.2020.05.027.

35. Sciomer, S., Moscucci, F., Magrì, D., Badagliacca, R., Piccirillo, G. and Agostoni, P. (2020). SARS-CoV-2 spread in Northern Italy: what about the pollution role?, *Environ. Monit. Assess.*, **192**, pp. 2–4. https://doi.org/10.1007/s10661-020-08317-y.

36. Setti, L., Passarini, F.,De Gennaro, G., Barbieri, P., Perrone, M.G., Borelli, M., Palmisani, J., Di Gilioc, A., Torboli, V., Fontana, F., Clemente, L., Pallavicini, A., Ruscio, M., Piscitelli, P. and Miani, A. (2020). SARS-Cov-2RNA found on particulate matter of Bergamo in Northern Italy: first evidence, *Environ. Res.*, **188**, p. 109754. https://doi.org/ 10.1016/j.envres.2020.109754.

37. Sharma, S., Zhang, M., Anshika, Gao, J., Zhang, H. and Kota, S. H. (2020). Effect of restricted emissions during COVID-19 on air quality in India, *Sci. Total Environ.*, **728**, p. 138878. https://doi.org/10.1016/ j.scitotenv.2020.138878.

38. Sicard, P., De Marco, A., Agathokleous, E., Feng, Z., Xu, X., Paoletti, E. and Calatayud, V. (2020). Amplified ozone pollution in cities during the COVID-19 lockdown, *Sci. Total Environ.*, **735**, p. 139542. https://doi.org/10.1016/j.scitotenv.2020.139542.

39. Singh, N., Tang, Y. and Ogunseitan, O. A. (2020). Environmentally sustainable management of used personal protective equipment, *Environ. Sci. Technol.*, **54**, pp. 8500–8502. https://doi.org/10.1021/acs.est.0c03022.

40. SNIS. Sistema Nacional de Informações sobre Saneamento (2018). *Diagnóstico dos serviços de água e esgotos.* http://www.snis.gov.br/ diagnostico-anual-agua-e-esgotos/diagnostico-dos-servicos-de-agua-e-esgotos-2018.

41. Sodré, F., Brandão, C. C. S., Vizzotto, C. S. and Maldanerc, A. O. (2020). Epidemiologia do esgoto como estratégia para monitoramento comunitário, mapeamento de focos emergentes e elaboração de sistemas de alerta rápido para COVID-19, *Quim. Nova*, **43**, pp. 515–519. http://dx.doi.org/10.21577/0100-4042.20170545.

42. Souza, L. P. S., Soares, A. F. S., Nunes, B. C. R., Costa, F. C. R. and Silva, L. F. M. (2020). Presença do novo coronavírus (SARS-CoV-2) nos esgotos sanitários: apontamentos para ações complementares de vigilância à saúde em tempos de pandemia, *Vigil. Sanit. Debate*, **8**, pp. 132–138. https://doi.org/10.22239/2317-269x.01624.

43. Suman, R., Javaid, M., Hallen, A. Vaishya, R., Bahl, S. and Nandan, D. (2020). Sustainability of coronavirus on different surfaces, *J. Clin. Exp. Hepatol.*, **10**, pp. 386–390. https://doi.org/10.1016/j.jceh.2020.04.020.

44. Wang, Y., Yuan, Y., Wang, Q., Liu, C., Zhi, Q. and Cao, J. (2020). Changes in air quality related to the control of coronavirus in China: implications for traffic and industrial emissions, *Sci. Total Environ.*, **731**, p. 139133. https://doi.org/10.1016/j.scitotenv.2020.139133.

45. World Health Organization (WHO) (2011). *Guidelines for Drinking-Water Quality*, **38**, pp. 104–108.

46. World Health Organization & United Nations Children's Fund (UNICEF) (2020). *Water, Sanitation, Hygiene and Waste Management for COVID-19: Technical Brief*, 03 March 2020. World Health Organization. https://apps.who.int/iris/handle/10665/331305. License: CC BY-NC-SA 3.0 IGO.

47. World Health Organization (WHO) (2020). *Air Pollution*. https://www.who.int/health-topics/air-pollution#tab=tab_1.

48. World Health Organization (WHO) (2020). Water, sanitation, hygiene, and waste management for SARS-CoV-2, the virus that causes COVID-19, *Interim Guidance*, pp. 1–21. WHO reference number: WHO/2019-nCoV/IPC_WASH/2020.4.

49. World Health Organization (WHO) (2020). Annual mean concentration of particulate matter of less than 2.5 microns of diameter (PM2.5) [ug/m3] in urban areas. https://www.who.int/data/gho/indicator-metadata-registry/imr-details/4674.

50. World Health Organization (WHO) (2020). Annual mean concentration of particulate matter of less than 10 microns of diameter (PM10) [ug/m3]. https://www.who.int/data/gho/indicator-metadata-registry/imr-details/1349>.

51. Wu, F., Xiao, A., Zhang, J., Gu, X., Lee, W., Kauffman, K., Hanage, W., Matus, M., Ghaeli, N., Endo, N., Duvallet, C., Moniz, K., Erickson, T., Chai, P., Thompson, J. and Alm, E. (2020). SARS-CoV-2 titers in wastewater are higher than expected from clinically confirmed cases, *medRxiv*, pp. 1–14. https://doi.org/10.1101/2020.04.05.20051540.

52. Wu, X., Nethery, R. C., Sabath, B. M., Braun, D. and Dominici, F. (2020). Exposure to air pollution and COVID-19 mortality in the United States, *medRxiv*, pp. 1–36. https://doi.org/10.1101/2020.04.05.20054502.

53. Xu, H., Yan, C., Fu, Q., Xiao, K., Yu, Y., Hand, D. and Cheng, J. (2020). Possible environmental effects on the spread of COVID-19 in China, *Sci. Total Environ.*, **731**, p. 139211. https://doi.org/10.1016/j.scitotenv.2020.139211.

54. Xu, Y., Li, X., Zhu, B., Liang, H., Fang, C., Gong, Y.,Guio, Q., Sun, X., Zhao, D., Shen, J., Zhang, H., Liu, H., Xia, H., Tang, J., Zhang, K. and Gong, S. (2020). Characteristics of pediatric SARS-CoV-2 infection and potential evidence for persistent fecal viral shedding, *Nat. Med.*, **26**, pp. 502–505. https://doi.org/10.1038/s41591-020-0817-4.

55. Zhang, Z., Xue, T. and Jin, X. (2020). Effects of meteorological conditions and air pollution on COVID-19 transmission: evidence from 219 Chinese cities, *Sci. Total Environ.*, **741**, p. 140244. https://doi.org/10.1016/j.scitotenv.2020.140244.

Chapter 3

Health Hazards of COVID-19

Aline Belem Machado, Gabriela Zimmermann Prado Rodrigues, Jorge Henrique Burghausen, Günther Gehlen, and Daiane Bolzan Berlese

Feevale University, ERS-239, 2755, 93525-075, Novo Hamburgo, Rio Grande do Sul, Brazil

linebmachado@hotmail.com, gabizpr@gmail.com, jorgeburghausen@yahoo.com.br, guntherg@feevale.br, daianeb@feevale.br

3.1 Pathways of Entry of the Virus into the Human Body

In mid-December 2019, a severe acute respiratory syndrome (SARS) caused by coronavirus 2 (SARS-CoV-2) triggered in China caught the world's attention due to the rapid spread of the epidemic. In two months, the World Health Organization declared the outbreak as a public health emergency of international interest, as other countries reported more and more cases [1].

Clinical data suggest that older adults or those with chronic health problems are more prone to severe illness, including death. The pathogenesis of the disease involves the entry of the virus into the cell, recognition by the body's defense cells, and inflammatory

Living with COVID-19: Economics, Ethics, and Environmental Issues

Edited by Chaudhery Mustansar Hussain and Gustavo Marques da Costa

Copyright © 2022 Jenny Stanford Publishing Pte. Ltd.

ISBN 978-981-4877-78-7 (Hardcover), 978-1-003-16828-7 (eBook)

www.jennystanford.com

immune response; however, this response can be influenced by and altered through mutations in the viral genome and even individual and ethnic variations among the hosts [2]. For example, the angiotensin-2-converting enzyme (ACE) serves as a receptor for SARS-Cov-2 in the human body and also acts as an effective modulator in lung injury, but it has been shown that its levels of expression and activity are altered under different conditions, as in individuals with diabetes [3], hypertension [4], kidney [5] and cardiovascular [6] disease, and smokers [7].

The ACE counterpart, ACE2, also serves as a gateway for the virus in the cell and is expressed as a membrane-bound protein by epithelial cells in various human tissues, such as lung, intestine, heart, kidney, and oral mucosa [8, 9]. After contact with ACE2, a transmembrane serine protease plays a crucial role in activating the fusion of the virus with the cell membrane, and the Furin protease mediates the proteolysis of the S2 subunit of the spike (S) protein (a unique feature for SARS-CoV-2) [8, 10]. The infected cell has a reduction in ACE2 levels, leading to synergistic effects in the induction of pulmonary fibrosis [8].

Then, SARS-CoV-2 (COVID-19) binds to ACE2 by its (S) protein and allows COVID-19 to enter and infect the cell. In order for the virus to complete cell entry after this initial process, the (S) protein must be initiated by an enzyme called protease (TMPRSS2) [11]. After the virus enters the host cell and unwinds, the genome is transcribed and then translated (the process occurs in the plasma membranes). For such processes, in addition to RNA polymerase, RNA helicase, and RNA-dependent protease activity, it has been reported that for the coronavirus there is the activity of a variety of RNA processing enzymes that are not (or extremely rarely) found in other viruses of RNA (putative sequence-specific endoribonuclease, exoribonuclease 3′ to 5′, methyltransferase 2′-O-ribose, 1P-ribose 1′-phosphatase ADP, and in a subset of group 2 coronavirus) [11, 12].

Therefore, it is possible to realize that after entering the cell, SARS-CoV-2 has the help of numerous proteins to perform its viral function, which will be addressed later in this chapter.

3.2 Proteins Involved

The new coronavirus (SARS-CoV-2) is classified as a member of the genus *Betacoronavirus*, is characterized by a single-stranded RNA genome with a positive sense, and is encoded by a relatively low number of proteins, being classified as structural and nonstructural. Among the main structural proteins are S glycoproteins, envelope (E) proteins, membrane (M) proteins, and nucleocapsid (NC) proteins [13, 14].

It is already reported that the first interaction that triggers the SARS-CoV-2 virus disease in the human body, at the molecular level, is the binding of the (S) protein to ACE2 [15]. The S1 and S2 receptor-binding domain of the (S) protein binds to the ACE2 receptor, as the viral envelope binds to the membrane and becomes internalized [16]. The (S) protein gene encodes a 150 KDa glycoprotein with 1255 amino acids. This protein is able to mediate membrane fusion and induce neutralizing antibodies in the host, which increases the chances of antibodies against the (S) protein and increases the chances of early detection and neutralization infection [17].

The (NC) protein is usually involved in the process of replication, transcription, and packaging of the virus genome and can hamper the reproductive cycle of the infected cell. This protein is the most abundant in coronaviruses, has great immunogenic capacity, and has a conserved amino acid sequence, making the protein promising for the development of vaccines and diagnostic studies [17, 18].

Similar to proteins S and NC, protein E is involved in many stages of virus infection in the host. This protein has 72 amino acids and can be found in monomeric and homopentameric forms. In previous studies, up to 20 copies of the protein were found and showed that it plays a crucial role in the beginning of the infection [19]. This protein is located inside the secretory pathways in the interspace between the endoplasmic reticulum and the Golgi apparatus and is also considered highly immunogenic, which attracts the attention of researchers to the development of antigens for immunodiagnostics and in the development of vaccines [19, 20].

The (E) protein is also involved in several stages of the virus infection and is located within the secretory pathways in the interspace between the endoplasmic reticulum and the Golgi apparatus [21]. During the replication cycle, it occurs abundantly within the infected cell, but only a small portion is incorporated into the virion envelope [22]. Recombinant coronaviruses without the (E) protein exhibit significantly reduced viral titers, impaired viral maturation, or incompetent production propagation progeny [23].

3.3 Effects on Human Health

The complement system is an old system that contributes to the innate immune response, and that includes cleavage proteins that play an important role in the defense against microorganisms, including viruses [24]. Viral inactivation carried out by the complement cascade involves the action of macrophages, through the capture of viruses and removal of their coating, resulting in the impossibility of binding with their cell receptors and viral lysis [25]. The involvement of this system in the specific case of COVID-19 results in the hyperactivation of complement components, including C5a in sera and C5b-9 in the lungs [26]. Therefore, this pathway is generally associated with the pathogenesis of SARS-CoV-2, with depositions of these and other complements observed in pulmonary and circulating autopsies in severe cases of COVID-19.

These immune reactions in severe COVID-19 can characterize the cytokine storm that is associated with undesirable clinical-pathological consequences. The cytokine storm is an uncontrolled release of cytokines, observed in some infectious and noninfectious diseases, leading to a condition of hyperinflammation in the host [24, 27], resulting in aggravated cases of this disease. About 10% of the patients with severe COVID-19 will experience lung injury, acute respiratory distress syndrome (ARDS), and multiple organ involvement within 8 to 14 days after the onset of their disease [28].

Then, the disease caused by the new coronavirus (SARS-CoV-2) is classified as an acute respiratory infection, having a high rate of transmission through close contact with infected individuals or by respiratory droplets present in the air. A person's first contact with the new corona virus is associated with mild symptoms, such as dry cough, malaise, tiredness, runny nose, and fever, usually present in other respiratory diseases already known to medicine, and also with gastrointestinal symptoms, including fever, cough, fatigue, and diarrhea. These symptoms occur during the virus incubation period, and it is during this period that SARS-CoV-2 benefits from multiplication in the host, mainly in the cells of the respiratory system [16, 29].

COVID-19 patients can be divided into four categories on the basis of their clinical manifestations: mild, common, severe, and critical [29]. In all cases, fever and cough are the most common symptoms, while diarrhea and vomiting are among the rarest [30]. Among symptomatic patients, pneumonia is the most common complication, followed by ARDS and shock. Thrombocytopenia was detected in 5%–41.7% of the patients with COVID-19, especially in the most severe cases, in addition to coagulation disorders [29]. In addition, patients with severe disease and fatal outcomes show a decrease in the proportion of lymphocytes compared to nonsevere patients [31]. Reported thrombocytopenia is mainly derived from direct attack of hematopoietic/progenitor stem cells and damage to the lungs by autoantibodies and immune complexes and can result in disseminated intravascular coagulation and multiple organ dysfunction syndrome, which lead to the deaths of critically ill patients [29].

Airborne transmission is linked to ACE2 receptors. A diagnosis of infection by blood count will show lymphopenia and neutrophilia without other significant abnormalities, and the treatment indicated by doctors is for the relief and reduction of symptoms [32]. In more advanced stages of the disease, inflammation and viral multiplication infect the lungs, where patients can develop viral pneumonia. And in more severe cases, hypoxia occurs, this being the stage where most patients need to be hospitalized, receiving specific treatments according to their clinical conditions. If hypoxia occurs, patients are likely to need mechanical ventilation, and corticosteroids are administered and performed judiciously on the basis of a medical evaluation [32].

The same authors [32] explain that in the third stage of the disease, classified as severe, where extrapulmonary systemic hyperinflammation develops in the organisms, a small portion of infected patients may have a decrease in the number of auxiliary T cells, suppressors, and regulators.

In addition to the physical damage that SARS-CoV-2 can cause to infected people, negative mental health impacts are also present, both for infected people and those who have not had contact with the virus, due to the quarantine and social isolation situation, imposed to prevent the large-scale spread of the new coronavirus. Such circumstances are capable of triggering an increase in the number of people with depression, anxiety attacks, and psychological crises, among other negative emotions [33].

A study developed by Lau et al. [34], which evaluated the emotional conditions of a population affected by the epidemic of SARS in 2003, found an increase in mental health problems, with higher levels of pessimism and negative thoughts, among the population in view of the situation they were experiencing. A study by Wang et al. [33], which assessed the prevalence of anxiety and depression symptoms in the Chinese population in the initial period of the pandemic caused by COVID-19, found an increase in the levels of anxiety and depression in the research participants, especially in cases where family members were infected by the virus.

Some pre-existing comorbidities have demonstrated to be higher risk factors for worsening of COVID-19, such as diabetes mellitus (DM), hypertension, and coronary heart disease [35, 36]. Patients with COVID-19 and pre-existing DM demonstrated to have more alterations in laboratory markers and worse prognosis when compared to COVID-19 patients without DM [37]. In DM, type 1 or type 2, and hypertension the expression of ACE2 is increased in patients treated with ACE inhibitors and angiotensin II type-I receptor blockers (ARBs), which results in an upregulation of ACE2 [35]. The study by Fang et al. [35] suggests that the use of these drugs consequently increases the expression of ACE2 in patients with DM, which in turn can facilitate the infection caused by COVID-19. Therefore, they hypothesize that patients with DM and hypertension who receive this type of treatment have an increased risk for developing severe and fatal COVID-19. However, this hypothesis is not proven in any experimental study and should be cautiously and carefully taken into consideration, since ACE inhibitors and ARBs are the most potent drugs against cardiovascular disease caused by hypertension [38].

A study performed by Guo and collaborators [39] analyzed if diabetes is a risk factor for COVID-19. They evaluated 174 patients with proven SARS-CoV-2 admitted to a hospital in Wuhan. Of these patients, 37 (21.2%) had diabetes and 43 (24.7%) had hypertension. A comparison of patients with diabetes and those without diabetes showed the following: patients with diabetes were older (61 vs. 32), presented with more nausea and vomiting (16.7% vs. 0%), and had higher mortality (16% vs. 0%). They concluded that SARS-CoV-2 pneumonia is more severe in patients with diabetes than those without this comorbidity. Therefore, diabetes patients should receive more intensive attention regarding the COVID-19 infection.

Significant alterations in blood exams have demonstrated that COVID-19 patients with comorbidities are at higher risk of tissue injury related to enzyme release, excessive uncontrolled inflammation responses, and hypercoagulable state, which can result in a poorer prognosis of COVID-19. This study highlights that comorbidities can have an impact on the progression and prognosis of COVID-19 [39]. However, a study performed by Zhu and collaborators [40] highlights the importance of patients with COVID-19 and DM having well-controlled glycemia, which results in a marked improvement in these patients [40].

References

1. Raza, S. S. and Khan, M. A. (2020). Mesenchymal stem cells: a new front emerge in COVID19 treatment: mesenchymal stem cells therapy for SARS-CoV2 viral infection, *Cytotherapy*, doi:10.1016/j.jcyt.2020.07.002.

2. Gupta, R. and Misra, A. (2020). COVID19 in South Asians/Asian Indians: heterogeneity of data and implications for pathophysiology and research, *Diabetes Res. Clin. Pract.*, **165**, p. 108267.

3. Lin, M., Gao, P., Zhao, T., He, L., Li, M., Li, Y., Shui, H. and Wu, X. (2016). Calcitriol regulates angiotensin-converting enzyme and angiotensin converting-enzyme 2 in diabetic kidney disease, *Mol. Biol. Rep.*, **43**(5), pp. 397–406.

4. Cui, C., Xu, P., Li, G., Qiao, Y., Han, W., Geng, C., Liao, D., Yang, M., Chen, D. and Jiang, P. (2019). Vitamin D receptor activation regulates microglia polarization and oxidative stress in spontaneously hypertensive rats and angiotensin II-exposed microglial cells: role of renin-angiotensin system, *Redox Biol.*, **26**, p. 101295.

5. Velkoska, E., Patel, S. K., Griggs, K., Pickering, R. J., Tikellis, C. and Burrell, L. M. (2015). Short-term treatment with diminazene aceturate ameliorates the reduction in kidney ACE2 activity in rats with subtotal nephrectomy, *PLoS One*, **10**(3), p. e0118758.

6. Ramchand, J., Patel, S. K., Srivastava, P. M., Farouque, O. and Burrell, L. M. (2018). Elevated plasma angiotensin converting enzyme 2 activity is an independent predictor of major adverse cardiac events in patients with obstructive coronary artery disease, *PLoS One*, **13**(6), p. e0198144.

7. Cai, G. (2020). Bulk and single-cell transcriptomics identify tobacco-use disparity in lung gene expression of ACE2, the receptor of 2019-nCov, *MedRxiv*, doi:https://doi.org/10.1101/2020.02.05.20020107.

8. Ghafouri-Fard, S., Noroozi, R., Omrani, M. D., Branicki, W., Pośpiech, E., Sayad, A., Pyrc, K., Łabaj, P., Vafaee, R., Taheri, M. and Sanak, M. (2020). Angiotensin converting enzyme: a review on expression profile and its association with human disorders with special focus on SARS-CoV-2 infection, *Vasc. Pharmacol.*, **130**, p. 106680.

9. Xu, H. and OuYang, Q. (2019). A new neighborhood structure and its fast evaluation strategy in using iterated local search to solve single machine scheduling, *Proc. 2019 9th Int. Workshop Comput. Sci. Eng.*, pp. 1–5.

10. Heurich, A., Hofmann-Winkler, H., Gierer, S., Liepold, T., Jahn, O. and Pöhlmann, S. (2014). TMPRSS2 and ADAM17 cleave ACE2 differentially and only proteolysis by TMPRSS2 augments entry driven by the severe acute respiratory syndrome coronavirus spike protein, *J. Virol.*, **88**(2), pp. 1293–1307.

11. Mousavizadeh, L. and Ghasemi, S. (2020). Genotype and phenotype of COVID-19: their roles in pathogenesis, *J. Microbiol., Immunol. Infect.*, in press.

12. Ziebuhr, J. (2005). The coronavirus replicase. In *Coronavirus Replication and Reverse Genetics*. Springer, Berlin, Heidelberg, pp. 57–94.

13. Chen, Y., Liu, Q. and Guo, D. (2020). Emerging coronaviruses: genome structure, replication, and pathogenesis, *J. Med. Virol.*, **92**(4), pp. 418–423.

14. Tilocca, B., Soggiu, A., Sanguinetti, M., Musella, V., Britti, D., Bonizzi, L., Urbani, A. and Roncada, P. (2020). Comparative computational analysis

of SARS-CoV-2 nucleocapsid protein epitopes in taxonomically related coronaviruses, *Microbes Infect.*, **22**(4–5), pp. 188–194.

15. Williamson, G. and Kerimi, A. (2020). Testing of natural products in clinical trials targeting the SARS-CoV-2 (COVID-19) Viral Spike Protein-Angiotensin Converting Enzyme-2 (ACE2) interaction, *Biochem. Pharmacol.*, **178**, p. 114123.

16. Wan, Y., Shang, J., Graham, R., Baric, R. S. and Li, F. (2020). Receptor recognition by the novel coronavirus from Wuhan: an analysis based on decade-long structural studies of SARS coronavirus. *J. Virol.*, **94**(7), p. e00127-20.

17. Chang, M. S., Lu, Y. T., Ho, S. T., Wu, C. C., Wei, T. Y., Chen, C. J., Hsu, Y. T., Chu, P. C., Chen, C. H., Chu, J. M., Jan, Y. L., Hung, C. C., Fan, C. C. and Yang, Y. C. (2004). Antibody detection of SARS-CoV spike and nucleocapsid protein, *Biochem. Biophys. Res. Commun.*, **314**(4), pp. 931–936.

18. Guo, L., Ren, L., Yang, S., Xiao, M., Chang, D., Yang, F., Cruz, C. S. D., Wang, Y., Wu, C., Xiao, Y., Zhang, L., Han, L., Dang, S., Xu, Y., Yang, Q. W., Xu, S. Y., Zhu, H. D., Xu, Y. C., Jin, Q., Sharma, L., Wang, L. and Wang, J. (2020). Profiling early humoral response to diagnose novel coronavirus disease (COVID-19), *Clin. Infect. Dis.*, **71**(15), pp. 778–785.

19. Stodola, J. K., Dubois, G., Le Coupanec, A., Desforges, M. and Talbot, P. J. (2018). The OC43 human coronavirus envelope protein is critical for infectious virus production and propagation in neuronal cells and is a determinant of neurovirulence and CNS pathology, *Virology*, **515**, pp. 134–149.

20. Bianchi, M., Benvenuto, D., Giovanetti, M., Angeletti, S., Ciccozzi, M. and Pascarella, S. (2020). Sars-CoV-2 envelope and membrane proteins: structural differences linked to virus characteristics?, *BioMed Res. Int.*, **2020**, p. 4389089.

21. Tilocca, B., Soggiu, A., Sanguinetti, M., Babini, G., De Maio, F., Britti, D., Zecconi, A., Bonizzi, L., Urbani, A. and Roncada, P. (2020). Immunoinformatic analysis of the SARS-CoV-2 envelope protein as a strategy to assess cross-protection against COVID-19, *Microbes Infect.*, **22**(4–5), pp. 182–187.

22. Schoeman, D. and Fielding, B. C. (2019). Coronavirus envelope protein: current knowledge, *Virol. J.*, **16**(1), pp. 1–22.

23. DeDiego, M. L., Álvarez, E., Almazán, F., Rejas, M. T., Lamirande, E., Roberts, A., Shieh, W. J., Zaki, S. R., Subbarao, K. and Enjuanes, L. (2007). A severe acute respiratory syndrome coronavirus that lacks the E gene is attenuated in vitro and in vivo, *J. Virol.*, **81**(4), pp. 1701–1713.

24. Mahmudpour, M., Roozbeh, J., Keshavarz, M., Farrokhi, S. and Nabipour, I. (2020). COVID-19 cytokine storm: the anger of inflammation, *Cytokine*, **133**, p. 155151.

25. Spear, G. T., Hart, M., Olinger, G. G., Hashemi, F. B. and Saifuddin, M. (2001). The role of the complement system in virus infections, *Curr. Top Microbiol. Immunol.*, **260**, pp. 229–246.

26. Jiang, Y., Zhao, G., Song, N., Li, P., Chen, Y., Guo, Y., Li, J., Du, L., Jiang, S., Gui, R., Sun, S. and Zhou, Y. (2018). Blockade of the C5a–C5aR axis alleviates lung damage in hDPP4-transgenic mice infected with MERS-CoV, *Emerg. Microbes Infect.*, **7**(1), pp. 1–12.

27. Tisoncik, J. R., Korth, M. J., Simmons, C. P., Farrar, J., Martin, T. R. and Katze, M. G. (2012). Into the eye of the cytokine storm, *Microbiol. Mol. Biol. Rev.*, **76**(1), pp. 16–32.

28. Lan, J., Ge, J., Yu, J., Shan, S., Zhou, H., Fan, S., Zhang, Q., Shi, X., Wang, Q., Zhang, L. and Wang, X. (2020). Structure of the SARS-CoV-2 spike receptor-binding domain bound to the ACE2 receptor, *Nature*, **581**(7807), pp. 215–220.

29. Zhang, Y., Jiao, Y., Li, Z., Yang, M. and Ye, J. (2020). Mechanisms involved in the development of thrombocytopenia in patients with COVID-19, *Thromb. Res.*, **193**, pp. 110–115.

30. Guan, W. J., Ni, Z. Y., Hu, Y., Liang, W. H., Ou, C. Q., He, J. X., Liu, L., Shan, H., Lei, C. I., Hui, D. S. C., Du, B., Li, L. J., Zeng, G., Yuen, K. Y., Chen, R. C., Tang, C. L., Wang, T., Chen, P. Y., Xiang, J., Li, S. Y., W., L. L., Liang, Z. J., Peng, Y. X., Wei, L., Liu, Y., Hu, Y. H., Peng, P., Wang, J. J., Qiu, S. Q., Luo, J., Ye, C. J., Zhu, S. Y. and Zhong., N. S. (2020). Clinical characteristics of coronavirus disease 2019 in China, *New Engl. J. Med.*, **382**(18), pp. 1708–1720.

31. Qu, R., Ling, Y., Zhang, Y. H. Z., Wei, L. Y., Chen, X., Li, X. M., Liu, X. Y., Liu, H. M., Guo, Z., Ren, H. and Wang, Q. (2020). Platelet-to-lymphocyte ratio is associated with prognosis in patients with coronavirus disease-19, *J. Med. Virol.*, **92**(9), pp. 1533–1541.

32. Siddiqi, H. K. and Mehra, M. R. (2020). COVID-19 illness in native and immunosuppressed states: a clinical–therapeutic staging proposal, *J. Heart Lung Transplant.*, **39**(5), p. 405.

33. Wang, Z. H., Yang, H. L., Yang, Y. Q., Liu, D., Li, Z. H., Zhang, X. R., Zhang, Y. J., Shen, D., Chen, P. L., Song, W. Q., Wang, X. M., Wu, X. B., Yang, X. F. and Mao, C. (2020). Prevalence of anxiety and depression symptom, and the demands for psychological knowledge and interventions in college students during COVID-19 epidemic: a large cross-sectional study, *J. Affect. Disord.*, **275**, pp. 188–193.

34. Lau, J. T., Yang, X., Tsui, H. Y., Pang, E. and Wing, Y. K. (2006). Positive mental health-related impacts of the SARS epidemic on the general public in Hong Kong and their associations with other negative impacts, *J. Infect.*, **53**(2), pp. 114–124.

35. Fang, L., Karakiulakis, G. and Roth, M. (2020). Are patients with hypertension and diabetes mellitus at increased risk for COVID-19 infection?, *Lancet. Respir. Med.*, **8**(4), p. e21.

36. Singh, A. K., Gupta, R., Ghosh, A. and Misra, A. (2020). Diabetes in COVID-19: prevalence, pathophysiology, prognosis and practical considerations, *Diabetes Metab. Syndr. : Clin. Res. Rev.*, **14**(4), pp. 303–310.

37. Zhang, Y., Cui, Y., Shen, M., Zhang, J., Liu, B., Dai, M., Chen, L., Han, D., Fan, Y., Zeng, Y., Li, W., Lin, F., Li, S., Chen, X. and Pan, P. (2020). Association of diabetes mellitus with disease severity and prognosis in COVID-19: a retrospective cohort study, *Diabetes Res. Clin. Pract.*, **165**, p. 108227.

38. Simone, G. and Mancusi, C. (2020). Speculation is not evidence: antihypertensive therapy and COVID-19, *Eur. Heart J.-Cardiovasc. Pharmacother.*, **6**(3), pp. 133–134.

39. Guo, W., Li, M., Dong, Y., Zhou, H., Zhang, Z., Tian, C., Qin, R., Wang, H., Shen, Y., Du, K., Zhao, L., Fan, H., Luo, S. and Hu, D. (2020). Diabetes is a risk factor for the progression and prognosis of COVID-19, *Diabetes/Metab. Res. Rev.*, p. e3319.

40. Zhu, L., She, Z. G., Cheng, X., Qin, J. J., Zhang, X. J., Cai, J., Lei, F., Wang, H., Xie, J., Wang, W., Li, H., Zhang, P., Song, X., Chen, X., Xiang, M., Zhang, C., Bai, L., Xiang, D., Chen, M. M., Liu, Y., Yan, Y., Liu, M., Mao, W., Zou, J., Liu, L., Chen, G., Luo, P., Xiao, B., Zhang, C., Zhang, Z., Lu, Z., Wang, J., Lu, H., Xia, X., Wang, D., Liao, X., Peng, G., Ye P., Yang, J., Yuan, Y., Huang, X., Guo, J., Zhang, B. H. and Li, H. (2020). Association of blood glucose control and outcomes in patients with COVID-19 and pre-existing type 2 diabetes, *Cell Metab.*, **31**(6), pp. 1068–1077.e3.

Chapter 4

Personal Protective Equipment and Coronavirus Disease

**Daniela Patrícia Freire Bonfim, Bruno de Araújo Lima,
Tayanna Cristina Passos Pereira, Marília Sonego,
Alessandro Estarque de Oliveira, Vádila Giovana Guerra, and
Mônica Lopes Aguiar**

*Federal University of São Carlos, Rodovia Washington Luís, km 235,
13565-905, São Carlos, SP, Brazil*
mlaguiar@ufscar.br

Coronavirus disease (COVID-19) is caused by severe acute respiratory syndrome coronavirus 2 (SARS-CoV-2), which presents a clinical picture ranging from asymptomatic infections to severe respiratory conditions. The new coronavirus, as it is called, was discovered on December 31, 2019, after cases were registered in China, and until August 17, 2020, about 21,756 million cases and 771,635 deaths from COVID-19 had been registered worldwide, according to World Health Organization (WHO) data. Although the transmission of COVID-19 occurs mainly via droplets during close contact with contaminated people or contaminated surfaces, a recent study has shown that SARS-CoV-2 remains viable in aerosols for many hours. Despite the efforts of the population and the agencies responsible for epidemiological control on a global scale,

Living with COVID-19: Economics, Ethics, and Environmental Issues
Edited by Chaudhery Mustansar Hussain and Gustavo Marques da Costa
Copyright © 2022 Jenny Stanford Publishing Pte. Ltd.
ISBN 978-981-4877-78-7 (Hardcover), 978-1-003-16828-7 (eBook)
www.jennystanford.com

the spread of SARS-CoV-2 is ongoing, creating a public health crisis and impacting the population worldwide. In this context, this chapter presents an updated scenario on the use of personal protective equipment (PPE) in relation to the combat and prevention of COVID-19 and the transmission of bioaerosols and a review of current regulations for the production, use, and certification of PPE. In addition, the chapter presents the importance of using PPE in disease prevention, especially using masks, on the basis of studies of effectiveness in previous epidemics, which allow us to modify and adapt fabrics and polymeric materials for making homemade masks.

4.1 Importance of Using PPE in Disease Prevention

The World Health Organization (WHO) declared a global health emergency associated with COVID-19 on January 30, 2020, and subsequently declared it to be a pandemic, on March 12, 2020, due to the global spread. COVID-19, first detected in Wuhan, Hubei Province, China, has caused concern by expanding rapidly in China and the rest of the world [87]. Coronavirus disease is caused by severe acute respiratory syndrome coronavirus 2 (SARS-CoV-2), a betacoronavirus, similar to the coronavirus of severe acute respiratory syndrome (SARS-CoV), already known to the medical community. Seasonal alpha- and betacoronaviruses cause common colds, croup, and bronchitis, and it is known that the modes of transmission of coronaviruses in humans are similar, which may be by droplets, contact, and, sometimes, air routes [58]. Science explains that the air route is a significant route of virus infection, so it is extremely important that authorities recognize the reality that the virus spreads through air and recommend that appropriate control measures be implemented to prevent the spread of SARS-CoV-2 [64].

In response to this concern and the rapid growth in the number of cases, the discussion regarding the feasibility of using personal protective equipment (PPE), especially related to protection against droplets and aerosols, has become a worldwide matter, mainly among the bodies responsible for maintaining health. PPE is needed in the current scenario, and mainly for the protection of employees who deal with COVID-19 patients. It is estimated that 40% of the health-care workforce will be infected and removed from the workforce due to exposure to the virus, mainly through respiratory droplets emitted by patients [6]. Several studies report that the use of PPE can significantly reduce the infection risk associated with the care of patients with coronavirus disease. As long as there is little evidence regarding which PPE provides the best protection, training in dressing and exchange, simulation, and face-to-face instructions is likely to be beneficial [80]. The main types of PPE used are medical masks, respirators (mainly N95/FFP2), face shields, goggles, gloves, and gowns, in association with basic hygiene measures, mainly of the hands, and they are classified according to the type of precaution required.

There are several different levels of PPE, including standard, contact, droplet, and airborne. Standard precautions include hand hygiene; respiratory hygiene with a cough tag; proper patient place-ment; and handling/cleaning of equipment, devices, environment, and laundry; as well as following safety procedures for sharps. Contact precautions are used when transmission occurs through direct contact with an infected individual or with contaminated body fluids or items. Droplet precautions are initiated in cases where the infection is spread through direct contact with contaminated droplets—talking, sneezing, or coughing. Airborne precautions are necessary for airborne diseases, as smaller droplets or pathogenic particles can travel further and remain suspended in the air for longer than the bigger droplets, requiring a separate set of droplet precautionary recommendations. Airborne diseases, such as COVID-19, tuberculosis, chickenpox, and measles, require patients to stay in negative pressure rooms, for example. The Centers for Disease Control and Prevention (CDC) gives different recommendations for PPE for each of these precaution levels [7]. It is important that the protocols recommended for the use and removal of PPE are correctly followed by the entire medical community. The protection offered by the equipment is related to correct utilization since the most common errors, such as insufficient PPE, incorrect apron removal, touching nonsterile surfaces, and not using the face mask protection, represent a violation of biosafety and lead to contamination [65, 69].

Recommendations for the use of PPE by professionals caring for suspected and/or confirmed COVID-19 patients are well established. Among the PPE, the mask has been given a lot of prominence, but its isolated use does not provide full protection. To be effective, it is essential to follow other measures, such as using other PPE (glasses or face shields, gloves, medical gowns, aprons, etc.), following correct and regular hand hygiene, isolating suspected and/or confirmed patients, and monitoring asymptomatic patients and staff for early identification and isolation of suspected cases. There are specific protocols for the medical and nursing staff in relation to the correct measures for the treatment of infected patients, for isolated areas for the treatment of COVID-19, and also for family members who want to go to hospitals or in cases of home isolation. In the fight against COVID-19 the WHO makes some recommendations for the use of PPE [89]. These rules vary by location, such as hospital and residential settings, and by type of personnel, such as workers and patients. The main differences in the recommendations can be seen in Table 4.1.

Most studies on previous respiratory virus epidemics to date suggest surgical masks are not inferior compared with N95 respirators. A strong protective effect of both masks has been in fact demonstrated, especially when used in combination with other protective measures, like hand washing, eye protection, gowns, and gloves [14].

The use of facemasks and respirators for the protection of health-care workers (HCWs) received renewed interest following the 2009 influenza pandemic and emerging infectious diseases, such as avian influenza, Middle East respiratory syndrome coronavirus (also known as MERS coronavirus), and Ebola virus. Historically, various types of cloth/cotton masks (referred to hereafter as "cloth masks") have been used to protect HCWs. Disposable medical/surgical masks (referred to hereafter as "medical masks") were introduced into health care in the mid-nineteenth century, followed later by respirators [60]. Before that, in the seventeenth-century Europe, doctors who cared for victims of the plague wore a cape that covered them from head to toe and wore a mask like a long bird's beak. Even

Table 4.1 WHO recommendations for PPE use against COVID-19 in hospital and home ambiences

Facility	Locality	Personnel	Activities	Recommendations
Hospital care	Patient room/ward	Health-care workers	Providing direct care to COVID-19 patients in the absence of aerosol generating procedures	• Wear a medical mask. • Wear a gown. • Wear gloves. • Wear eye protection (goggles or a face shield). • Perform hand hygiene (PHH).
			Providing direct care to COVID-19 patients in settings where aerosol generating procedures are frequent	• Use respirator N95, FFP2, or FFP3 standard or equivalent. • Wear a gown. • Wear gloves. • Wear eye protection. • Wear an apron. • PHH.

(Contd.)

Table 4.1 *(Contd.)*

Facility	Locality	Personnel	Activities	Recommendations
		Cleaners	Entering rooms with COVID-19 patients	• Wear a medical mask. • Wear a gown. • Wear heavy-duty gloves. • Wear eye protection (if there is risk of organic materials or chemical splash). • Wear closed work shoes. • PHH.
	Traffic area without patients (cafeteria, corridors)	Visitors	Entering rooms with COVID-19 patients	• Maintain a physical distance of at least 1 m. • Wear a medical mask. • Wear a gown. • Wear gloves. • PHH.
		Staff	Doing any activity that does not include contact with COVID-19 patients	• Maintain a physical distance of at least 1 m. • PPE is not required. • PHH.

Home care	Patients with COVID-19 symptoms	Doing any	• Maintain a physical distance of at least 1 m. • Wear a medical mask if tolerated. • Perform hand and respiratory hygiene.
	Caregivers	Entering a patient's room but not providing direct care or assistance	• Maintain a physical distance of at least 1 m. • Wear a medical mask. • PHH.
	Caregivers	Providing direct care to or handling stool, urine, or waste from COVID-19 patients at home	• Wear gloves. • Wear a medical mask. • Wear an apron. • PHH.
	Health-care workers	Providing direct care or assistance to COVID-19 patients	• Wear gloves. • Wear a medical mask. • Wear a gown. • wear eye protection.

Source: Adapted from Ref. [89].

though at the time the use of these protective clothing had no effect, doctors had already thinking about ways of protecting themselves from pandemic diseases. Subsequently, these early measures served as a basis for studies and for the development of PPEs [10].

Meta-analysis of studies in healthy health-care providers (on whom most studies have been performed) has indicated a strong protective value provided by both surgical masks and N95 respirators [68] against clinical and respiratory virus infection. Case control data from the 2003 SARS epidemic suggests a strong protective value provided by mask use by community members in public spaces, on the order of 70% [33]. This understanding is essential to convey that the use of only masks does not give sufficient protection to fight the new coronavirus and to ensure that PPE can be used rationally, making certain that there is no PPE scarcity in situations where its use is indispensable [62]. To facilitate the population's access to auxiliary products in the prevention of contagion and evaluated from the point of view of the risk-benefit ratio so favorable to patients and the population in general, several exceptional and temporary measures have been established as a way to minimize the current health problem for the public.

As has been reported, the coronavirus can spread through droplets suspended in the air when infected people speak, cough, or sneeze, and these droplets can be reduced with the use of non-professional masks. These masks act as physical barriers, reducing exposure and the risk of infection for the general population. It is important to highlight that professional masks (industrialized medical surgical material) must be kept exclusively for use by health professionals and contaminated patients, where nonprofessional masks are useless [20, 64].

In summary, the benefit of routine use of face masks by the general public during the COVID-19 pandemic remains uncertain. However, several studies in progress suggest a possible strong potential benefit for the almost universal adoption of weakly effective homemade masks that can be synergized with, but cannot replace, other control and mitigation measures. Thus, it is important that masks not be viewed as an alternative to but as a complement to other public health control measures (including nonpharmaceutical interventions, such as social distancing and self-isolation) [58].

Table 4.2 The transmission routes of some infectious agents

Pathogen (disease)	Aerosol transmission	Droplet transmission
Bordetella pertussis (whooping cough)	No	Yes
Influenza virus (influenza)	Yes*	Yes
Adenovirus (flu)	No	Yes
Rhinovirus (flu)	Yes*	Yes
Mycoplasma pneumoniae (pneumonia)	No	Yes
Coronavirus (SARS-CoV) (severe acute respiratory syndrome)	No	Yes
Group A streptococcus (scarlet fever)	No	Yes
Neisseria meningitidis (meningitis)	No	Yes
Mycobacterium tuberculosis (tuberculosis)	Yes	No
Rubeola virus (measles)	Yes	No
Varicella-zoster virus (chickenpox)	Yes	No
Variola virus (smallpox)	Yes*	Yes
Coronavirus (SARS-CoV-2; COVID-19)	Yes*	Yes

*There is some evidence of transmission.
Source: Adapted from Ref. [77].

4.2 Transmission of Bioaerosols

Bioaerosols are airborne biological particles with sizes varying from 10 μm to 50 nm [49]. They include bacteria, viruses, fungi, and even DNA fragments that can come in contact with the skin or enter the human body by the respiratory tract during inhalation, causing allergies, toxic reactions, and infections [49]. Larger particles (>5 μm), known as droplets, can also contain infectious pathogens and transmit infections. Moreover, droplet nuclei (<5 μm) can be formed after the evaporation of droplets [77]. Table 4.2 shows some infectious diseases transmitted by aerosols and droplets.

This differentiation based on the transmission routes of aerosols and droplets is essential for recommending the most appropriate PPE [23], as can be seen in Table 4.3.

Infectious droplets and aerosols expelled by patients during breathing, speaking, coughing, and sneezing (Table 4.4) are suspended in the air and able to contaminate healthy people around them. People can also be infected by touching surfaces contaminated with infected particles, termed fomites [31, 63, 91].

Table 4.3 PPE recommended depending on the transmission route of the infectious agent

Transmission route	When to use	PPE
Contact	>2 m from patient	Gloves and apron
Droplet	Within 2 m from patient	Gloves, apron, fluid-resistant surgical mask, and goggles/visor
Aerosol	Aerosol generation procedure	Gloves, fluid-repellent long-sleeved gown, goggles/visor, and respirators

Source: Adapted from Ref. [23].

Table 4.4 The number of droplets and aerosols expelled by humans during regular activities

Activity	Number of droplets	Aerosols	Initial velocity (m/s)
Normal breathing	A few	Some	1
Talking	A few to a few dozen	Mostly	5
Coughing	A few hundred	Mostly	10
Sneezing	A few hundred thousand to a few million	Mostly	20–50

Source: Adapted from Refs. [31, 63, 91].

Many factors affect the spread of particles in air, including their size, their initial velocity, relative humidity, and ventilation [77, 91]. Large particles fall to the ground quickly; however, they can travel more than 2 m (coughing) or 6 m (sneezing) due to higher initial velocities, as represented in Fig. 4.1. Small droplets evaporate quickly, whereas aerosols may remain suspended in air for many hours, depending on the Brownian motion, electrical forces, thermal gradients, and turbulent diffusion [31]. These particulate dynamics models are probabilistic, and other factors influence the transmission of infectious disease [63, 77].

The concentration of pathogens in bioaerosols and droplets affects the respiratory infection transmission risk. For instance, in susceptible guinea pigs, the inhalation of only one droplet enclosing

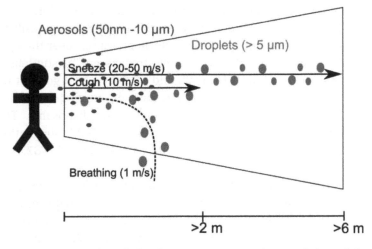

Figure 4.1 Aerosol and droplet movement in the air (adapted from Ref. [91]).

three tubercle bacilli can result in conversion tuberculin testing and macroscopic granuloma [61, 84]. The viral load needed for the transmission of COVID-19 is still unknown; however, many studies associated a higher viral load and more severe symptoms of the disease [83].

4.3 Standards Currently in Force for PPE

In addition to recommending the protective equipment to be used in each situation, the WHO also recommends norms and standards that each type of equipment must meet. The following are the recommendations for the main PPE [89]:

- Face shield: It must be made of transparent plastic in order to provide good visibility for the user and the patient. It should have an adjustable band for fastening so it can be adapted to the user's head and be worn comfortably, completely covering the sides and the length of the face. It may be reusable (after cleaning) or disposable. The standards suggested by the WHO for the face shield are EU PPE Regulation 2016/425, EN 166, and ANSI/ISEA Z87.1 or an equivalent set of standards.

- Protective goggles: They must seal well with the skin of the face, have a flexible polyvinyl chloride (PVC) frame to easily fit all contours of the face with uniform pressure, cover the eyes and the surrounding areas, have transparent plastic lenses with fog-resistant treatments and scratches, be a good fit on the user's head so as not to come loose during clinical activity, and may be reusable (after cleaning) or disposable. The WHO-suggested standards for goggles are EU PPE Regulation 2016/425 Category III, EN 166, and ANSI/ISEA Z87.1 or equivalent.
- Gloves: Gloves can be for examination (nitrile, powder-free, and nonsterile, with a minimum thickness of 0.05 mm) or surgical (latex, sterile, and powder-free, with a minimum thickness of 0.1 mm and long cuffs). The WHO-suggested standards for examination gloves are EU MDD (directive) 93/42/EEC Class I, EU PPE Regulation 2016/425 Category III, FDA Class 1, EN 455, EN 374, ASTM D6319, or an equivalent set of standards. For surgical gloves, the suggested standards are EU MDD (directive) 93/42/EEC Class IIa, EU PPE Regulation 2016/425 Category III, FDA Class 1, EN 455, ASTM D3577, EN ISO 11607, and sterility according to USP or set standards equivalent.
- Gown: The dresses can be examination or surgical, the only difference being the sterility of the second. They must be disposable and be long enough to cover up to the middle of the calf. The WHO-suggested standards for examination gowns are EU MDD (directive) 93/42/EEC Class I, EU PPE Regulation 2016/425 Category III, FDA Class 1, and EN 13795 any performance level or AAMI PB70 all levels or ASTM F3352. For surgical gowns, the suggested standards are EU MDD (directive) 93/42/EEC Class IIa, EU PPE Regulation 2016/425 Category III, FDA Class 2 or equivalent, EN 13795 any performance level or AAMI PB70 all levels, and ASTM F2407.
- Apron: The heavy-duty apron must be straight with a bib. The apron must be made of 100% polyester with a PVC coating, 100% PVC, 100% rubber, or other fluid-resistant coating

material or it must be waterproof, with a handle sewn for neck and back attachment. The WHO-acceptable standards for heavy-duty aprons are EN ISO 13688, EN 14126-B and partial body protection (EN 136034 or EN 14605), and EN 343 for water and breathability or equivalent.

- Medical masks: They must have good breathability with the internal and external sides clearly identified. The standards for medical masks suggested by the WHO are EN 14683 and ASTM 2100 of any level of classification for patients. For HCWs, the suggested standards are EN 14683 Type II, ASTM 2100 minimum Level 1, FDA Class 2, EU PPE Regulation 2016/425 Category III, and EU MDD (directive) 93/42/EEC Class I or an equivalent set of standards.

- Respirator N95/FFP2 or higher: It must have good breathability and a design that does not collapse with the mouth. The respirator standards suggested by the WHO are EN 149 for minimum FFP2, NIOSH 42 CRF 84 for minimum N95, FDA Class 2, EU PPE Regulation 2016/425 Category III, and EU MDD (directive) 93/42/EEC Class I or an equivalent set standards.

The standards and regulations suggested by the WHO for PPE use are basically European or North American. These standards standardize the dimensions of the protective equipment, from the body size of the equipment, the size of strips and fixtures, and construction materials to the performance characteristics of the equipment in the protection of the individual. For example, according to ASTM D6319 [2], the gloves must meet the sterility requirements, comply with the absence of holes, have consistent physical dimensions, have acceptable physical characteristics, have a powder residue limit of 2 mg, and have a maximum recommended powder limit of 10 mg/dm^2. According to ASTM F2407 [4], the gown must be biocompatible, comply with the level of sterility guarantee, and comply with the requirements for Class 1 flammable items, and if it contains latex, it should be reported and the physical properties should be tested. In addition, it must pass the material conditioning test. These tests are interrelated.

The main characteristics of the standards for respiratory protection equipment are described in more detail next since the main route of transmission of COVID-19 is the respiratory route.

4.3.1 Respiratory PPEs

Respiratory PPE, like masks and respirators, is intended to protect the user's airway against a harmful atmosphere. The respiratory protection devices used to prevent the transmission of infectious diseases can be divided into the following groups: surgical masks and respirators (FFP2/N95 and FFP3/N98) for HCWs and patients (if possible) and cloth masks (homemade) for the general population, since commercial ones are scarce.

4.3.1.1 Masks

Surgical masks protect the mouth, nose, and respiratory tract against droplets and particles. They provide good permeability to air and steam, resulting in reasonable comfort during use. Surgical masks are nonreusable and should be discarded after any change in activity, damage, or contamination by any body fluid. These kinds of masks retain particles and droplets emitted by the user and do not protect the user against external pathogens. Therefore, they are used to prevent disease transmission by the user when he or she speaks, breaths, coughs, or sneezes.

These masks are regulated by EN 14683 [78] and ASTM F2100 [3]. EN 14683 is a European standard that describes the construction and performance requirements and test methods for medical face masks. The masks specified in this standard are classified as Type I and Type II depending on bacterial resistance, and Type II can be divided according to their resistance to splashes (Type IIR). According to this standard, the medical face mask should contain a filter layer between the layers of tissue and should be fitted over the nose, mouth and complain. ASTM F2100 [2019] [3] is a North American standard that consists of specifying the performance of the materials used in the masks. Thus, this standard provides performance classification for a variety of materials used in mask construction.

The specified properties represent the sector characterizing the performance of the material, but they do not include all aspects. The materials for medical face masks that are within this standard are classified on the basis of performance in various tests and can be Level 1, Level 2, and Level 3. Both standards are very similar since they use methodologies with small variations. The main requirements for these standards are described in Table 4.5.

Most surgical masks have three main layers, described in Table 4.3. Although polypropylene (PP) is the most common polymer, polystyrene, polyethylene, polycarbonate, and polyester can also be used to produce surgical masks.

The inner layer, described in Table 4.6, is essential for moisture absorption, whereas the outer layer is designed to prevent droplet passage from the user to the atmosphere. The middle layer is, in fact, the filtering layer, which is nonwoven and with very thin fibers, produced by the melt-blowing process. In this process, when the melted polymer reaches the spinning head of the extruder, it is drawn into filaments (1–8 μm, typically) by a high-speed/temperature airflow, forming the nonwoven fabric [71]. Moreover, electrostatic finishing can be adopted to improve filtration efficiency, especially for smaller particles [47].

4.3.1.2 Respirators

Differently from surgical masks, the respirators protect the respiratory tract against particles, droplets, and aerosols. They protect the user against infectious agents and also prevent their spread and contagion. Their efficacy mostly depends on their facial fit, needed for sealing, filtration efficiency of solid and liquid particles, and breathing resistance.

Respirators can be disposable or not and should be changed after each activity, when damaged or contaminated, or when breathing becomes difficult.

In Europe, the minimum requirements of each class of respirators (FFP1, FFP2, and FFP3) are dictated by the EN 149 standard, the main tests of which are described in Table 4.7. The protection levels appointed as FFP2 and FFP3 are equivalent to the Americans N95 and N98, respectively [36].

Table 4.5 EN 14683 and ASTM F2100 main requirements for surgical masks

Test	EN 14683				ASTM F2100		
	Type I	Type II	Type IIR	Level 1	Level 2	Level 3
Bacterial filtration efficiency (%)	≥ 95	≥ 98	≥ 98	≥ 95	≥ 98	≥ 98
Differential pressure (mmH₂O)/cm²)	<3	<3	<5	<3	<3	<5
Submicron particulate filtration at 0.1 μm (%)	Not required	Not required	Not required	≥ 95	≥ 98	≥ 98
Splash resistance/synthetic blood resistance (mmHg pass result)	Not required	Not required	120 (16 kPa)	80	120	160
Flame spread	Not required	Not required	Not required	Class 1	Class 1	Class 1
Microbial cleanliness (CFU/g)	≤ 30	≤ 30	≤ 30	Not required	Not required	Not required

Source: Adapted from Ref. [34].

Table 4.6 Common layers found in surgical masks

Inner layer	Nonwoven PP spunbond (18–25 g/m^2)
Filtration layer	Nonwoven PP melt-blown (25 g/m^2) with an electrostatic finish
Outer layer	Nonwoven PP spunbond (18–25 g/m^2)

Source: Adapted from Ref. [36].

Table 4.7 Requirements for respirators according to the EN 149 standard

Class	Internal leak (%)	Particle penetration (% max.)		Breathing resistance (mbar)	
		NaCl 95 L/min.	Paraffin oil 95 L/min.	Inhalation 95 L/min.	Exhalation 160 L/min.
FFP1	22	20	20	2.1	3
FFP2	8	6	6	2.4	3
FFP3	2	1	1	3	3

Source: Adapted from Ref. [36].

An FFP2 or FFP3 respirator usually contains a filter layer between two support layers. The filter layer includes a nonwoven mixture of fine fibers and larger resilient fibers, which form a compact interfelted mass with small pores [46]. The fine fibers, responsible for the barrier properties, can be made of PVC, polyamide, or PP. The resilient fibers (rayon, acrylic, PP, polyethylene, polyamide, or polysulfone) avoid the excessive formation of fine fibers clusters. The filter layer can include 4–20% w/w of fine fibers, depending on its diameter [46]. Other filter layers can be made by melt-blow and receive an electrostatic treatment [36]. The support layers are made of nonwoven fabric with resilient fibers (rayon, acrylic, PP, polyethylene, polyamide, or polysulfone) with a density between 20 and 50 g/m^2.

Thus, the FFP2/FFP3 respirators can also have exhalation valves, which improve the wear comfort but do not filter the exhaled air. Therefore, they do not protect people around the user against contamination. Table 4.8 gives the different types of protection provided by masks and respirators.

Specifically for COVID-19 pandemic, the recommendations of the European Safety Federation according to the communication

Table 4.8 Protection by surgical masks and respirators against infectious organisms

Respiratory protective device	User protection against infectious organisms (one-way protection)	Prevention of emission of infectious organisms (two-way protection)
Surgical mask	Yes	No
FFP2/FFP3 respirators without exhalation valves	Yes	Yes
FFP2/FFP3 respirators with exhalation valves	Yes	No

European Commission after "concerns following the appeal by many (health) authorities to produce 'artisanal' masks at home or any possible production site" are surgical masks EN 14683-Type II or superior and respirators EN149-FFP2 or superior, just like WHO recommendations.

The PFF2/N95 respirators have a minimum filtration efficiency of 94% at 0.3 μm particle diameter. However, it is not clear whether these respirators show high filtration efficiency against biological aerosols smaller than that, like SARS-CoV-2, which have a size between 0.06 and 0.14 μm [92]. A recent study conducted by 3M tested the filtration efficiency of five different respirators against aerosols containing two types of influenza viruses (H1N1 and H5N1; size 0.08–0.12 μm). For all respirators tested, the filtration efficiency for the virus was about 1%–2% higher than for the most penetrating particle size (in this case about 0.4 μm) [1].

4.3.1.3 Homemade masks

The worldwide scarcity of protective masks and respirators during the COVID-19 pandemic promoted the use of homemade masks or cloth masks to diminish the spread of the virus. Although the decision is controversial, an increasing number of countries have been asking their citizens to wear homemade masks in public settings during this pandemic [18, 85]. At the same time, many household fabrics have been tested as filters in the search for the best homemade mask [27, 37, 47, 67, 74].

According to Rengasamy et al. [74], the penetration level (inverse of filtration efficiency) of cloth masks and improvised materials (sweatshirt, T-shirt, towel, and scarf) of polydisperse NaCl aerosol at 5.5 cm/s face velocity is in the rage of 74%–90%, much higher than the 0.12% measured for N95 respirators. For monodisperse aerosol particles in the range of 20–1000 nm, the fabrics showed penetration levels between 40% and 97%. Such values agree with previous measurements of penetration levels of 54% (particle size of 400 nm) and 59% (particle size of 1000 nm) at 1.5 cm/s [24]. Although the penetration levels measured for these household materials are high, they are close to the 51%–89% range obtained by some surgical masks at the same face velocity. Among the improvised materials tested, the sweatshirt showed the lowest penetration level against polydisperse and monodisperse (<60 nm) aerosols [74]. The authors also argue that filtration performance depends on the characteristics of the fiber more than the fabric composition [74].

The filtration efficiency and pressure drop across a wide range of household materials can be seen in Table 4.9. The tests were conducted with two microbial aerosols, *Bacillus atrophaeus* (0.95–1.25 μm) and Bacteriophage MS2 (MCIMB10108) (23 nm) [27]. Considering the high filtration efficiency and low pressure drop, 100% cotton T-shirts and pillowcases are the best options for homemade masks. However, as surgical masks showed the best filtration performance, improvised masks should only be used as a protective device as the last possible alternative.

Homemade masks of another variety were tested using optical scattering measurements, which compare the intensity of light dispersion by droplets before and after passing through the mask [37]. In these experiments, the best filtration performance was achieved by homemade masks with a higher number of layers, woven fabrics with less porosity, and fabrics with a high cotton percentage.

An increasing the number of fabric layers, that is, a larger mask thickness, also contributed to a better filtration performance of homemade masks [42, 67]. Double-layered masks and masks folded four times showed filtration efficiencies (particle size range 0.3–10 μm) 1.7–4.6 and 2.3–6.8 times higher than their single-layered version [42].

Table 4.9 Filtration efficiency of household materials against microbial aerosols and pressure drop

Material	*Bacillus atrophaeus*		Bacteriophage MS2			
	Mean filtration efficiency (%)	Standard deviation	Mean filtration efficiency (%)	Standard deviation	Pressure drop	Standard deviation
100% cotton T-shirt	69.42	10.53	50.85	16.81	4.29	0.07
Scarf	62.30	4.44	48.87	19.77	4.36	0.19
Tea towel	83.24	7.81	72.46	22.6	7.23	0.96
Pillowcase	61.28	4.91	57.13	10.55	3.88	0.03
Antimicrobial pillowcase	65.62	7.64	68.9	7.44	6.11	0.35
Surgical mask	96.35	0.68	89.52	2.65	5.23	0.15
Vacuum cleaner bag	94.35	0.74	85.95	1.55	10.18	0.32
Cotton mix	74.60	11.17	70.24	0.08	6.18	0.48
Linen	60	11.18	61.67	2.41	4.5	0.19
Silk	58	2.75	54.32	29.49	4.57	0.31

Source: Adapted from Ref. [27].

Penetration of particles (P) decreases exponentially with filter thickness (L), according to Eq. 4.1, for a particular particle size [40].

$$P = e^{-\beta L},\qquad (4.1)$$

where β depends on particle size, face velocity, fiber diameter, and filter solidity.

Penetration decreases with filter thickness since the particles lose velocity and momentum, being more easily captured when they pass through the medium. The pressure drop is directly proportional to the filter thickness at a given face velocity, as the multilayered medium is made of filters in series in which air resistance must be added [40]. Therefore, multilayered homemade masks are a simple strategy to increase filtration efficiency without severely compromising pressure drop.

Another strategy to improve the filtration efficiency of home-made masks is to combine mechanical and electrostatic-based filtration, like cotton-silk, cotton-chiffon, and cotton-flannel multi-layered masks. Konda et al. [47] made an attempt to analyze the performance of different fabrics used as cloth masks, besides N95 respirators and surgical masks, using NaCl particles from 10 nm to 10 μm in air at traveling at 12 and 32 ft^3/min. The authors evaluated cloth masks of cotton quilt consisting of two 120 threads-per-inch (TPI) cotton sheets enclosing an $\sim$0.5 cm thick cotton batting, 80 TPI quilters cotton, and 600 TPI cotton, besides different combinations of layers of chiffon (1 and 2 layers), natural silk (1, 2, and 4 layers), and flannel and combinations of these materials. The results showed that a single layer of fabric provided 5% to 80% of collection efficiency for particles of sizes less than 300 nm and 5% to 95% for particles greater than 300 nm, while the combinations of different fabrics provided efficiencies above 80% and 90% for particles less and higher than 300 nm, respectively; the most closed net of threads provided the highest efficiency, but none of the cloth masks surpassed the efficiency of the N95 mask, of 95% efficiency to particles higher than 300 nm. Although there is no report on the fiber size or even the porosity of the filter media, this work presented interesting results concerning the effect of leakage through the space between the mask and the face, which led to a decrease of 60% in the collection efficiency for particles larger than

Table 4.10   Recommendation when washing cloth masks

Recommended procedures	Observations
Using the washing machine	The mask can be included with regular laundry, using laundry detergent and the warmest temperature.
Washing by hand	The mask must be submerged in a bleach solution for 5 min.
Drying	The mask should be dried in the highest heat setting or in direct sunlight.

Source: Adapted from Ref. [25].

300 nm. The same trend was observed by Cho et al. [21] studying N95 masks and by Lin et al. [52] studying different decontamination methods—including bleach, ethanol, and autoclave—in N95 and nonwoven commercial masks.

One advantage of cloth masks for the general public is that they are washable and reusable [16, 25]. The CDC recommended that masks must be washed (Table 4.10) after each use [25].

In fact, decontamination is required to ensure that a mask continues protecting the wearer from the pathogens, but there can be risks in this process and great care must be taken. Neupane et al. [66] evaluated the effect of multiple cycles of washing and drying and also the effect of stretching on the structure and performance of commercial cloth masks that had original PM_{10} efficiencies of 63% to 84%, and surgical masks, with original efficiency of 94% for PM_{10}. The results showed that the mean pore size varied between the cloth masks (81 to 461 μm) and the mask with the smallest pore size had the highest efficiency, which was not better than that of the surgical mask (whose pore size was not measured). However, both the stretching and the cycles of washing and drying increased the pore size of the cloth masks and subsequently reduced the efficiency for PM_{10} from ∼63% to ∼20%. There was no information on the fiber size.

Additionally, Liu et al. [53] focused on the effect of talking and face washing on the contamination of different masks used by surgeons in an operating room, reporting that the number of colony-forming units (CFUs) in the masks were significantly lower in the case of no speaking and the mask with the highest efficiency and the lowest porosity provided the best restraint against bacterial shedding from the user. The authors observed that face washing reduced the number of CFUs in the face of the user, but no significant variation was observed in the mask, which could lead to a risk of further contamination.

Boškoski et al. [14] reported an efficient method of decontamination of N95 masks and respirators from viral respiratory agents by highly energetic shortwave ultraviolet germicidal irradiation at 254 nm, but it requires careful consideration of the type of respirator and of the biological target. Luan and Ching [55] suggest making a face mask by combining a surgical mask and a cardiopulmonary resuscitation (CPR) mask, in which the main idea is to place fragments of the surgical mask in the CPR mask. These masks would be washable with easy-to-use liquid agents (using 75% alcohol solution or bleach), and after use the filter would be discarded and the mask reused. This means that if the surgical mask is cut into six samples, we can have at least six pieces of filter per piece of face mask [55].

The effectiveness of a homemade mask against aerosols/droplet infections greatly depends on a good facial fit, which prevents leakage from around the mask [27]. A great advantage of PFF2/N95 respirators against surgical masks is that the latter have a fit requirement ensuring the minimum leakage of particles around the mask. Several mask prototypes have been proposed to improve the facial fit [16, 26]. Figure 4.2 shows a prototype mask (size 4) that reached a fit factor of 67 when tested by the Portacount Plus

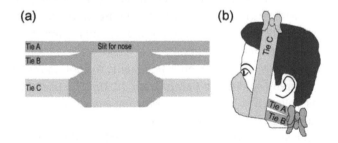

Figure 4.2 Homemade mask prototype tested by the Portacount Plus Respirator Fit Tester: (a) mask view and (b) proper use of the mask. Adapted from Ref. [26].

Respirator Fit Tester, which requires a minimum value of 100 for commercial N95 respirators [26].

4.4 Results/Effectiveness in Previous Epidemics

In view of the uncertainty regarding coronavirus disease, an analysis of the results of preventive measures and control effectiveness in the face of previous epidemics allows us to evaluate the use and development, mainly, of PPEs throughout history. During the bubonic plague in the Renaissance, some physicians used a beak-like mask, a coat covered in scented wax, hat, and gloves of goat leather when attending plague victims, a kind of primordial PPE [11]. The masks contained holes for breathing and perfume, which was intended to protect the physician from miasma, or "poisoned air." Although the costume has been famous since then, it was not effective against the bubonic plague, as fleas are the disease vector.

One of the first mentions of mask effectiveness against airborne transmission of diseases was during the great Manchurian pneumonic plague epidemic in 1910–1911 and 1920–1921 [57]. The head of the antiplague efforts, Dr. Wu Lien-Teh, made the HCWs wear cotton and gauze masks as a way to mitigate disease transmission [48]. Wu reported a low infection rate and mortality among physicians (mortality of 5% in 1910–1911 and 9% in 1920–1921) [48, 51]. Sanitary attendants had a mortality of 19% in the first outbreak and 43% in the second outbreak. The high degree of contact with patients, the lack of training, and the frequently improper use of masks were mentioned as causes for the higher mortality among the attendants.

In 1918, Capps [17] reported experiments to contain respiratory infections among soldiers in Camp Grant, IL, US. The use of the face mask was believed to be the most efficient measure to isolate the patients and decrease disease transmission.

In the last year of World War I, facial masks were largely adopted by HCWs and the general public to combat the Spanish influenza, the first of two pandemics caused by the H1N1 influenza A virus. Quarantine for those infected, disinfection/hygiene measures, closing places of public gathering (schools, church, commercial establishments), and mandatory use of gauze masks for citizens were measures adopted in many places, especially in the United States [12]. In the US city of Tucson-Arizona, the failure to use a mask in public places could lead to imprisonment, which caused many arrests during the period. Many people preferred to disregard the mask ordinance and take the risk of finding a police officer, but all had "handy masks for an emergency" [56]. However, milder and late public health interventions were taken in different US cities, for example, in Philadelphia and Washington, causing considerable variation in mortality rates in different cities [12]. By looking at the weekly mortality data reported in 16 cities during the period, it was possible to estimate the effect of different health interventions using an epidemic model [12]. The model showed that the interventions applied could attenuate total mortality by perhaps 10%–30%, thus having a moderate protective impact, mostly because the measures were introduced too late and revoked too early. Transmission rate reductions on the order of 30%–50% were achieved in San Francisco, St. Louis, Milwaukee, and Kansas City, where the measures were most effective [12]. The 1918–1919 Spanish Influenza pandemic had many similarities to the COVID-19, including health system collapse, scarcity of masks, economic crisis, and public criticism. This previous experience can be instructive in leading to actions and interventions during this current recent health crisis.

The use of PPE to constrain contagious diseases like tuberculosis, Ebola, SARS, and influenza has been investigated [43, 61, 68, 73]. However, it must be stated that proving PPE effectiveness in interrupting infection transmission is not easy, especially during the stressful periods of epidemics. Bias and uncertainty come from many factors: small sample size, comparison of heterogeneous trials, and self-reported clinical outcomes, among others. The most reliable conclusion comes from a systematic review of homogeneous randomized controlled clinical trials, which are scarce. A systematic review of homogeneous cohort and case-controlled studies is good and can be done frequently.

Table 4.11   Meta-analysis from case-control studies on PPE use to prevent severe respiratory syndrome (SARS)

PPE	Odds ratio	95% confidence interval	Number needed to treat (%)	95% confidence interval
Surgical masks	0.32	0.25–0.4	6	4.54–8.03
N95 respirators	0.09	0.03–0.3	3	2.37–4.06
Gloves	0.43	0.29–0.65	5	4.15–15.41
Gowns	0.23	0.14–0.37	5	2.66–4.97

Source: Adapted from Ref. [43].

A meta-analysis with six case-control studies carried out between 2003 and 2005 evaluated the impact of wearing masks, gloves, and gown on interrupt the transmission of SARS [43]. Five studies used hospital cases whereas one selected case was of people with probable SARS reported to authorities in Hong Kong. The use of masks, N95 respirators, gloves, and gowns was found to be an effective protective measure, as can be checked in Table 4.11.

Another meta-analysis with two randomized controlled trials also confirmed the beneficial effect of wearing a surgical mask or N95 respirators. Masks and respirators are effective against clinical respiratory illness (risk ratio [RR] = 0.59; 95% confidence interval [CI]: 0.46–0.77) and influenza-like illness (RR = 0.34; 95% CI: 0.14–0.82) [68].

During the H1N1 influenza pandemic of 2009, many observational studies evaluated the use of respiratory PPE by HCWs against the virus [68]. In California, 21% of the workers in contact with influenza patients and without PPE contracted the disease, whereas none of the workers wearing masks or respirators got sick [41]. Similarly, in Hong Kong, the medical staff wearing surgical masks remained healthy while 1.5% of the workers without masks developed pH1N1 seroprevalence [19]. However, four cross-sectional studies in Japan and Thailand showed no association between the use of masks/respirators and pH1N1 infection [5, 22, 81, 86].

Most studies are concerned about the transmission of infectious diseases to HCWs. Differently, a cluster-randomized trial compared the self-reported use of surgical masks, use of nonfitted P2 masks, and no use of masks to prevent the influenza-like transmission in households [59]. The volunteers were 286 adults from 143 different houses who had been exposed to a child with a respiratory illness. The study concluded that adherent mask users had a relative reduction of 60%–80% in the daily risk of contracting a respiratory infection [59]. However, the adherence to mask use most of the time was less than 50%. The authors argue that in a more severe pandemic, the adherence to respiratory PPE may be higher.

The use of PPE had become emblematic during the Ebola epidemic in West Africa, starting in 2013. The Ebola virus is found in body fluids like blood, urine, sweat, vomitus, and stool that HCWs are likely to come in contact with when attending patients [32]. According to the WHO, between 2014 and 2015, about 881 HCWs contracted the Ebola virus and 513 of them died [88]. The PPE to be used when attending Ebola patients should cover all the skin (scrubs, footwear, coveralls, apron, gloves, face mask and visor, and headwear) and requires great skill during its removal, even under the supervision of a trained observer. For example, it is recommended that hand hygiene with alcohol be performed multiple times during PPE removal. Recently, a new solution for PPE, as well as new donning and doffing protocols, was proposed [73]. However, there is a lack of information regarding the effectiveness of the PPE against Ebola transmission.

Tuberculosis, caused by the bacteria *Mycobacterium tuberculosis*, is another endemic disease that has been plaguing human society for long. Although the disease has been almost eradicated in the first world countries, many tuberculosis outbreaks took place in the United States and Europe in the mid-1980s and early 1990s, resulting in new guidelines for preventing its transmission [45]. The prevalence of tuberculosis in human immunodeficiency virus coinfection, lapses in infection control practices, and the emergence of multidrug-resistant strains of tuberculosis contributed to the disease resurgence [30]. Its occupational risk for HCWs in hospitals with more than 200 tuberculosis admissions is about 1%–10% [61]. Surgical masks were previously recommended to prevent the expiration of droplets (1–5 μm) containing viable tubercle bacilli. However, such masks fail to block inhalation of the particle in this particle size range, and thus the use of N95 respirators is recommended in actualized protocols and guidelines, especially during aerosol-generation procedures [29, 45, 61]. However, in practice, such respiratory PPE are infrequently used by HCWs even during high-risk procedures, at least in developing countries [9, 72, 76]. The lack of knowledge and training, unavailability of PPE, and discomfort during use are pointed to as reasons for the meager use of respirators and masks [9, 72, 76].

During the coronavirus disease pandemic, the use of respiratory PPE has been extensively investigated by systematic reviews and meta-analysis of previous respiratory infectious disease reports [8, 15, 44, 50, 90]. Until now, the studies have been contradictory or inconclusive and there is a lack of strong evidence on the effectiveness of PPE against COVID-19 transmission [38]. However, waiting for perfect scientific evidence to take simple and potentially effective measures, such as the use of masks in public places, can cost many lives [38, 44, 70].

4.5 PPE Modifications to Combat SARS-CoV-2

During the COVID-19 pandemic, a series of supply chain issues, constant changes in PPE use policy, and higher demand for PPE have led to shortages in PPE, specifically N95 masks and face shields. Implementation of decontamination protocols has successfully allowed N95 mask reuse but requires masks to be unsoiled. Given the great need for PPE in the face of high demand, several studies have been reported, giving suggestions such as reuse and readapt techniques, as mentioned before, and printing of 3D materials [14, 35, 82].

The University of Nebraska Medical Center, Omaha, NE, US, has produced face shields using a combination of 3D printing and assembly with commonly available products. Its ability to rapidly manufacture commercially available desktop FDM printers combined with open source and readily available materials has enabled the creation of sufficient face shields to provide protection until other, more durable shields can be purchased. A simple but effective method of decontamination was also created and implemented, which allowed the reuse of facial masks using the average log10 reduction in colony counts for *Escherichia coli* ATCC 8937 and *Staphylococcus aureus* ATCC 25923 of the American Type Culture Collection (ATCC, Manassas, VA, US). As per information in this paper, the rapid production of this product by individuals with little or no 3D printing experience can be easily accomplished in times of urgent need [6].

In addition to these changes in existing PPE and reuse techniques, the use of various materials as possible raw materials for making masks and protective fabrics has been reported in the literature. Thus, several techniques for making filter media have been reported as promising for modifying and adapting both fabrics and polymeric materials for making PPE [79].

Liu and colleagues [54] have successfully electrospun a biodegradable silk fibroin/poly(lactic-*co*-glycolic acid)/graphene oxide (SF/PLGA/GO) microfiber to use as a protective fabric. The addition of graphene promoted an increase in mechanical resistance, a higher Young's modulus, and better thermal stability to satisfy the requirements of its application. Besides that, the small pore size of the mat can effectively block particulate pollutants and pathogenic agents present in the air. The larger surface area and pore volume of the carpet are adequate for breathability of the fiber. Thus, the manufactured SF/PLGA/GO microfiber mat presents exciting features, making this material an efficient protective fabric [54]. Another biodegradable electrospun material with antibacterial potential was reported in the literature by Almeida et al. [28]. Experimental results indicated that the cellulose acetate/cetylpyridinium bromide nanofibers present good permeability and high-efficiency filtration for aerosol nanoparticles (about 100%), which may include black carbon and the new coronavirus. This research provides information for future designs of internal air filters and filter media for face masks with renewable, nontoxic, biodegradable characteristics and also antibacterial potential [28].

Polyacrylonitrile/copper oxide (PAN/CuO) nanofibers have also been reported to have been successfully electrospun with varying concentrations of CuO to produce nonwoven and antibacterial structures. CuO was selected as an antibacterial agent due to its good antimicrobial properties as well as for its economical production when compared to that of other metallic nanoparticles. Addition of CuO nanoparticles transmitted strength to PAN nanofibers, whose PAN/CuO tensile strength increased significantly (8.43 MPa), in addition to improved air permeability. The authors concluded that CuO nanoparticles have potential for antimicrobial and structural applications, and they recommend PAN/CuO nanoparticles for antimicrobial respirator applications [39]. Bortolassi et al. [13] also studied the efficient removal of nanoparticles and the bactericidal action with nanofibers for air filtration applications. Filters with high filtration efficiency ($\sim$100%) and a high-quality factor ($\sim$0.05 Pa^{-1}) were obtained by adding Ag nanoparticles in different concentrations to PAN nanofibers. The resultant Ag/PAN nanofibers showed excellent antibacterial activity against 104 CFU/mL *E. coli* bacteria. This antimicrobial character is very promising in the current scenario, which allows us to infer that this filter medium may be adapted so that the virucidal capacity is also used [13].

Material in which nanofibers are used in loaded multilayers has also been reported in the literature as promising for the manufacture of respirators. According to the study, polyvinylidene fluoride loaded with six layers of nanofiber filter provides good personal protection against the airborne COVID-19 virus and pollution based on the N98 standard but is at least 10 times more breathable than a conventional N95 respirator. The authors also concluded that 10–400 nm environmental aerosols can be captured by this filter with and without charge, with the unloaded nanofiber filter mainly presenting diffusion and interception capture mechanisms. In addition, when nanofibers are loaded, dielectrophoresis further helps to capture aerosols; this is especially true for large aerosols >80 nm [75].

As reported in the literature, the use of filter media, mainly nanofibers, has great potential for the manufacture of protective fabrics, masks, and respirators. In addition to the possibility of exploring morphological characteristics of these fibers at the time of their manufacture, which are associated with high filtration efficiency along with low pressure drop, there is also a great option for the functionalization of these nanofibers, giving them a biocidal character [13, 28, 54].

4.6 Final Considerations and Perspectives

Unfortunately, COVID-19 has caused a very large number of deaths and infections in the past few months and there is still a high likelihood of new cases emerging even in regions where the pandemic has been brought under control. In this sense, because it is a common and invisible enemy, the maintenance of protection measures with a global reach is necessary and urgent. In addition to health professionals, responsible authorities should be encouraged to use PPE. To try to minimize the problem of PPE shortages, new production techniques must be continuously investigated. In the last few years, it was possible to develop nanomaterials by new technologies and new materials were created with most diverse applications in society, health, the environment, and industry due to the wide dissemination of nanoscience concepts and the rapid advance of nanotechnology. Among the new materials, micro- and nanofibers have excelled in air filtration, with the manufacture of highly efficient smart membranes for the collection of nanoparticles, mainly bioaerosols—they are better than the filters currently commercialized—and are a very promising technology for manufacturing masks and PPEs. The manufacture of homemade masks is also an excellent option for the general population and offers a satisfactory degree of protection, as demonstrated in research and also based on the results of effectiveness in previous epidemics, but it is necessary to create research-based standards for the use and manufacture of these masks so that effective commonly available materials are increasingly used. In this sense, what we hope is that this delicate moment of public health crisis will be quickly solved by agencies responsible for epidemiological control on a global scale and that the development of new materials will continue in order to prevent another collapse in public health.

References

1. 3M (2020). Respiratory protection for airborne exposures to biohazards. Technical Data Bulletin, p. 10.

2. American Society for Testing and Materials (2019). ASTM D6319: standard specification for nitrile examination gloves for medical application, *ASTM Standards*, pp. 1–4. https://doi.org/10.1520/D6319-19.2.

3. American Society for Testing and Materials (2019). ASTM F2100: standard specification for performance of materials used in medical face masks, *ASTM Standards*, **11**(2018), pp. 19–21. https://doi.org/10.1520/F2100-11.2.

4. American Society for Testing and Materials (2020). ASTM F2407: standard specification for surgical gowns intended for use in healthcare facilities, *ASTM Standards*, **06**(reapproved 2013), pp. 1–8. https://doi.org/10.1520/F2407-06R13E01.performance.

5. Ang, B., Poh, B. F., Win, M. K. and Chow, A. (2010). Surgical masks for protection of health care personnel against pandemic novel swine-origin influenza A (H1N1)-2009: results from an observational study, *Clin. Infect. Dis.*, **50**(7), pp. 1011–1014. https://doi.org/10.1086/651159.

6. Armijo, P. R., Markin, N. W., Nguyen, S., Ho, D. H., Ms, T. S. H., Lisco, S. J. and Schiller, A. M. (2020). 3D printing of face shields to meet the immediate need for PPE in an anesthesiology department during the COVID-19 pandemic, *Am. J. Infect. Control*, in press. https://doi.org/10.1016/j.ajic.2020.07.037.

7. Associates, W. A., Hospital, S. F. and Ct, H. (2020). Personal protective equipment (PPE) guidelines, adaptations and lessons during the COVID-19 pandemic, *Ethics Med. Public Health*, **14**. https://doi.org/10.1016/j.jemep.2020.100546.

8. Bartoszko, J. J., Farooqi, M. A. M., Alhazzani, W. and Loeb, M. (2020). Medical masks vs N95 respirators for preventing COVID-19 in healthcare workers: a systematic review and meta-analysis of randomized trials, *Influenza Other Respir. Viruses*, **14**(4), pp. 365–373. https://doi.org/10.1111/irv.12745.

9. Biscotto, C. R., Pedroso, E. R. P., Starling, C. E. F. and Roth, V. R. (2005). Evaluation of N95 respirator use as a tuberculosis control measure in a resource-limited setting, *Int. J. Tuberc. Lung Dis.*, **9**(5), pp. 545–549.

10. Blakemore, E. (2020). Why plague doctors wore those strange beaked masks. Retrieved August 9, 2020, from https://www.national

geographic.co.uk/history-and-civilisation/2020/03/why-plague-doctors-wore-those-strange-beaked-masks.

11. Blakemore, E. (2020). Why plague doctors wore those strange beaked masks. Retrieved July 31, 2020, from https://www.national geographic.com/history/reference/european-history/plague-doctors-beaked-masks-coronavirus/.

12. Bootsma, M. C. J. and Ferguson, N. M. (2007). The effect of public health measures on the 1918 influenza pandemic in U.S. cities, *Proc. Natl. Acad. Sci.*, **104**(18), pp. 7588–7593. https://doi.org/10.1073/pnas.0611071104.

13. Bortolassi, A. C. C., Nagarajan, S., de Araújo Lima, B., Guerra, V. G., Aguiar, M. L., Huon, V., Soussan, L., Cornu, D., Miele, P. and Bechelany, M. (2019). Efficient nanoparticles removal and bactericidal action of electrospun nanofibers membranes for air filtration, *Mater. Sci. Eng. C*, 102, pp. 718–729. https://doi.org/ 10.1016/j.msec.2019.04.094.

14. Boškoski, I., Gallo, C., Wallace, M. B. and Costamagna, G. (2020). COVID-19 pandemic and personal protective equipment shortage: protective efficacy comparing masks and scientific methods for respirator reuse, *Gastrointest. Endosc.*, **92**(3), pp. 519–523. https://doi.org/10.1016/j.gie.2020.04.048.

15. Brainard, J. S., Jones, N., Lake, I., Hooper, L. and Hunter, P. (2020). Face-masks and similar barriers to prevent respiratory illness such as COVID-19: a rapid systematic review, *MedRxiv*, https://doi.org/10.1101/2020.04.01.20049528.

16. Brazilian Association of Technical Standards (ABNT) (2020). *Prática recomendada: Máscaras de proteção respiratória para uso não profissional - Guia de requisitos básicos para métodos de ensaio, fabricação e uso*, Prática recomendada No. ABNT PR 1002, Brazil.

17. Capps, J. A. (1918). Measures for the prevention and control of respiratory infections in military camps, *J. Am. Med. Assoc.*, **71**(6), p. 448. https://doi.org/10.1001/jama.1918.26020320008010a.

18. CDC (2020). Coronavirus disease 2019 (COVID-19). Retrieved July 3, 2020, from https://www.cdc.gov/coronavirus/2019-ncov/prevent-getting-sick/diy-cloth-face-coverings.html.

19. Cheng, V. C. C., Tai, J. W. M., Wong, L. M. W., Chan, J. F. W., Li, I. W. S., To, K. K. W., Hung, I. F. N., Chan, K. H., Ho, P. L. and Yuen, K. Y. (2010). Prevention of nosocomial transmission of swine-origin pandemic influenza virus A/H1N1 by infection control bundle, *J. Hosp. Infect.*, **74**(3), pp. 271–277. https://doi.org/10.1016/j.jhin.2009.09.009.

20. Cheng, V. C. C., Mnurs, S. W., Frcpath, V. W. M. C., So, S. Y. C., Chen, J. H. K., Frcpath, S. S., To, K. K. W., Chan, J. F. W. and Hung, I. F. N. (2020). The role of community-wide wearing of face mask for control of coronavirus disease 2019 (COVID-19) epidemic due to SARS-CoV-2, *J. Infect.*, **2019**. https://doi.org/10.1016/j.jinf.2020.04.024.

21. Cho, D., Naydich, A., Frey, M. W. and Joo, Y. L. (2013). Further improvement of air filtration efficiency of cellulose filters coated with nanofibers via inclusion of electrostatically active nanoparticles, *Polymer*, **54**(9), pp. 2364–2372. https://doi.org/10.1016/j.polymer.2013.02.034.

22. Chokephaibulkit, K., Assanasen, S., Apisarnthanarak, A., Rongrungruang, Y., Kachintorn, K., Tuntiwattanapibul, Y., Judaeng, T. and Puthavathana, P. (2013). Seroprevalence of 2009 H1N1 virus infection and self-reported infection control practices among healthcare professionals following the first outbreak in Bangkok, Thailand, *Influenza Other Respir. Viruses*, **7**(3), pp. 359–363. https://doi.org/10.1111/irv.12016.

23. Cook, T. M. (2020). Personal protective equipment during the coronavirus disease (COVID) 2019 pandemic: a narrative review, *Anaesthesia*, **75**(7), 920–927. https://doi.org/10.1111/anae.15071.

24. Cooper, D. W., Hinds, W. C. and Price, J. M. (1983). Emergency respiratory protection with common materials, *Am. Ind. Hyg. Assoc. J.*, **44**(1), pp. 1–6. https://doi.org/10.1080/15298668391404275.

25. Coronavirus Disease 2019 (COVID-19): How to Wash Masks (2020). Retrieved August 1, 2020, from https://www.cdc.gov/coronavirus/2019-ncov/prevent-getting-sick/how-to-wash-cloth-face-coverings.html.

26. Dato, V. M., Hostler, D. and Hahn, M. E. (2006). Simple respiratory mask. *Emerging Infect. Dis.*, **12**, pp. 1033–1034.

27. Davies, A., Thompson, K.-A., Giri, K., Kafatos, G., Walker, J. and Bennett, A. (2013). Testing the efficacy of homemade masks: would they protect in an influenza pandemic?, *Disaster Med. Public Health Prep.*, **7**(4), pp. 413–418. https://doi.org/10.1017/dmp.2013.43.

28. de Almeida, D. S., Martins, L. D., Muniz, E. C., Rudke, A. P., Squizzato, R., Beal, A., de Souza, P. R., Freire Bonfim, D. P., Aguiar, M. L. and Gimenes, M. L. (2020). Biodegradable CA/CPB electrospun nanofibers for efficient retention of airborne nanoparticles, *Process Saf. Environ. Prot.*, **144**, pp. 177–185. https://doi.org/10.1016/j.psep.2020.07.024.

29. Diel, R., Nienhaus, A., Witte, P. and Ziegler, R. (2020). Protection of healthcare workers against transmission of *Mycobacterium tuberculosis* in hospitals: a review of the evidence, *ERJ Open Res.*, **6**(1), pp. 00317-02019. https://doi.org/10.1183/23120541.00317-2019.

30. Dooley, S. W., Jarvis, W. R., Marione, W. J. and Snider, D. E. (1992). Multidrug-resistant tuberculosis, *Ann. Intern. Med.*, **117**(3), pp. 257–259. https://doi.org/10.7326/0003-4819-117-3-257.

31. Duguid, J. P. (1946). The size and the duration of air-carriage of respiratory droplets and droplet-nuclei, *J. Hyg.*, **44**(6), pp. 471–479.

32. Edmond, M. B. (2014). Personal protective equipment, 2.

33. Eikenberry, S. E., Mancuso, M., Iboi, E., Phan, T., Eikenberry, K., Kuang, Y., Kostelich, E. and Gumel, A. B. (2020). To mask or not to mask: modeling the potential for face mask use by the general public to curtail the COVID-19 pandemic, *Infect. Dis. Modell.*, **5**, pp. 293–308. https://doi.org/10.1016/j.idm.2020.04.001.

34. EN14683 Harmonizes Bacterial Filtration, Nelson Labs (2014).

35. Erickson, M. M., Richardson, E. S., Hernandez, N. M., Ii, D. W. B., Gall, K., Fearis, P. and Rca, M. (2020). Helmet modification to PPE with 3D printing during the COVID-19 pandemic at Duke University Medical Center: a novel technique, *J. Arthroplasty*, **35**(7), pp. S23–S27. https://doi.org/10.1016/j.arth.2020.04.035.

36. Fangueiro, R., Ferreira, D., Silva, C., Silva, P. and Navarro, M. (2020). *Máscaras de proteção*. Fibrenamics intelligence.

37. Foschini, M., Monte, A. F., Mendes, A. C., Scarabucci, R. J., Maletta, A., Giuliani, C. D., Duarte, B. A. and Del-Claro, K. (2020). Aerosol blocking assessment by different types of fabrics for homemade respiratory masks: spectroscopy and imaging study (preprint), *medRxiv*, https://doi.org/10.1101/2020.05.26.20100529.

38. Greenhalgh, T., Schmid, M. B., Czypionka, T., Bassler, D. and Gruer, L. (2020). Face masks for the public during the COVID-19 crisis, *BMJ*, m1435. https://doi.org/10.1136/bmj.m1435.

39. Hashmi, M., Ullah, S. and Kim, I. S. (2019). Current research in biotechnology copper oxide (CuO) loaded polyacrylonitrile (PAN) nano fiber membranes for antimicrobial breath mask applications, *Curr. Res. Biotechnol.*, **1**, pp. 1–10. https://doi.org/10.1016/j.crbiot.2019.07.001.

40. Hinds, W. C. (2012). Chapter 9: Filtration. In *Aerosol Technology: Properties, Behavior, and Measurement of Airborne Particles* (2nd ed.), John Wiley & Sons.

41. Jaeger, J. L., Patel, M., Dharan, N., Hancock, K., Meites, E., Mattson, C., Gladden, M., Sugerman, D., Doshi, S., Blau, D., Harriman, K., Whaley, M., Sun, H., Ginsberg, M., Kao, A. S., Kriner, P., Lindstrom, S., Jain, S., Katz, J., Finelli, L., Olsen, S. J. and Kallen, A. J. (2011). Transmission of 2009 pandemic influenza A (H1N1) virus among healthcare personnel—

Southern California, 2009, *Infect. Control Hosp. Epidemiol.*, *32*(12), pp. 1149–1157. https://doi.org/10.1086/662709.

42. Jang, J. Y. and Kim, S. W. (2015). Evaluation of filtration performance efficiency of commercial cloth masks, *J. Environ. Health Sci.*, **41**(3), pp. 203–215. https://doi.org/10.5668/JEHS.2015.41.3.203.

43. Jefferson, T., Foxlee, R., Mar, C. Del, Dooley, L., Ferroni, E., Hewak, B., Prabhala, A., Nair, S. and Rivetti, A. (2008). Physical interventions to interrupt or reduce the spread of respiratory viruses: systematic review, *BMJ*, **336**(7635), pp. 77–80. https://doi.org/10.1136/bmj.39393.510347.BE.

44. Jefferson, T., Jones, M., Al Ansari, L. A., Bawazeer, G., Beller, E., Clark, J., Conly, J., Del Mar, C., Dooley, E., Ferroni, E., Glasziou, P., Hoffman, T., Thorning, S. and Van Driel, M. (2020). Physical interventions to interrupt or reduce the spread of respiratory viruses. Part 1 - Face masks, eye protection and person distancing: systematic review and meta-analysis (preprint), Public and Global Health.

45. Jensen, P. A., Lambert, L. A., Iademarco, M. F. and Ridzon, R. (2005). Guidelines for preventing the transmission of *Mycobacterium tuberculosis* in health-care settings, 2005, *MMWR, Recommendations and Reports*, **54**(RR-17), pp. 1–141.

46. Weeks, T. and Reimschussel, G. P. (1973). Disposable face respirato, US Patent 3,779,244.

47. Konda, A., Prakash, A., Moss, G. A., Schmoldt, M., Grant, G. D. and Guha, S. (2020). Aerosol filtration efficiency of common fabrics used in respiratory cloth masks, *ACS Nano*, **14**(5), pp. 6339–6347. https://doi.org/10.1021/acsnano.0c03252.

48. Kool, J. L. (2005). Risk of person-to-person transmission of pneumonic plague, *Clin. Infect. Dis.*, **40**(8), pp. 1166–1172. https://doi.org/10.1086/428617.

49. Lee, B. U. (2011). Life comes from the air: a short review on bioaerosol control, *Aerosol Air Qual. Res.*, **11**(7), pp. 921–927. https://doi.org/10.4209/aaqr.2011.06.0081.

50. Liang, M., Gao, L., Cheng, C., Zhou, Q., Uy, J. P., Heiner, K. and Sun, C. (2020). Efficacy of face mask in preventing respiratory virus transmission: a systematic review and meta-analysis, *Travel Med. Infect. Dis.*, p. 101751. https://doi.org/10.1016/j.tmaid.2020.101751.

51. Lien-Teh, W. (1926). *A Treatise on Pneumonic Plague*. Geneva: League of Nations. Health Organization.

52. Lin, T. H., Chen, C. C., Huang, S. H., Kuo, C. W., Lai, C. Y. and Lin, W. Y. (2017). Filter quality of electret masks in filtering 14.6–594 nm aerosol particles: Effects of five decontamination methods, *PLoS One*, **12**(10), pp. 1–15. https://doi.org/10.1371/journal.pone.0186217.

53. Liu, Zhiqing, Yu, D., Ge, Y., Wang, L., Zhang, J., Li, H., Liu, F. and Zhai, Z. (2019). Understanding the factors involved in determining the bioburdens of surgical masks, *Ann. Transl. Med.*, **7**(23), pp. 754–760. https://doi.org/10.21037/atm.2019.11.91.

54. Liu, Zulan, Shang, S., Chiu, K., Jiang, S., Dai, F., Hong, T., Polytechnic, K. and Kong, H. (2020). Fabrication of silk fibroin/poly (lactic-co-glycolic acid)/graphene oxide microfiber mat via electrospinning for protective fabric, *Mater. Sci. Eng. C*, **107**, p. 110308. https://doi.org/10.1016/j.msec.2019.110308.

55. Luan, P. T. and Ching, C. T. (2020). A reusable mask for coronavirus disease 2019 (COVID-19), *Arch. Med. Res.*, **2019**. https://doi.org/10.1016/j.arcmed.2020.04.001.

56. Luckingham, B. (1984). To mask or not to mask: a note on the 1918 Spanish influenza epidemic in Tucson, *J. Arizona Hist.*, **25**(2), pp. 191–204.

57. Lynteris, C. (2018). Plague masks: the visual emergence of anti-epidemic personal protection equipment, *Med. Anthropol.*, **37**(6), pp. 442–457. https://doi.org/10.1080/01459740.2017.1423072.

58. Macintyre, C. R. and Ahmad, A. (2020). A rapid systematic review of the efficacy of face masks and respirators against coronaviruses and other respiratory transmissible viruses for the community, healthcare workers and sick patients, *Int. J. Nurs. Stud.*, **108**, p. 103629. https://doi.org/10.1016/j.ijnurstu.2020.103629.

59. MacIntyre, C. R., Cauchemez, S., Dwyer, D. E., Seale, H., Cheung, P., Browne, G., Fasher, M., Wood, J., Gao, Z., Booy, R. and Ferguson, N. (2009). Face mask use and control of respiratory virus transmission in households, *Emerging Infect. Dis.*, **15**(2), pp. 233–241. https://doi.org/10.3201/eid1502.081166.

60. MacIntyre, C. R., Seale, H., Dung, T. C., Hien, N. T., Nga, P. T., Chughtai, A. A., Rahman, B., Dwyer, D. E. and Wang, Q. (2015). A cluster randomised trial of cloth masks compared with medical masks in healthcare workers, *BMJ Open*, **5**(4). https://doi.org/10.1136/bmjopen-2014-006577.

61. Menzies, D., Fanning, A., Yuan, L. and Fitzgerald, M. (1995). Tuberculosis among health care workers. *N. Engl. J. Med.*, **332**(2), p. 7.

62. Michael Klompas, Charles A. Morris, Julia Sinclair, Madelyn Pearson, E. S. S. (2020). Universal masking in hospitals in the COVID-19 era. *N. Engl. J. Med.*, **63**(1), pp. 1–3.

63. Morawska, L. (2005). Droplet fate in indoor environments, or can we prevent the spread of infection? In X. Yang, B. Zhao, & R. Zhao (eds.), *Indoor Air 2005: Proceedings of the 10th International Conference on Indoor Air Quality and Climate.* CD Rom: Tsinghua University Press, pp. 9–23.

64. Morawska, L. and Cao, J. (2020). Airborne transmission of SARS-CoV-2: the world, *Environ. Int.*, p. 105730. https://doi.org/10.1016/j.envint.2020.105730.

65. Muñoz-Leyva, F. and Niazi, A. U. (2020). Common breaches in biosafety during donning and doffing of protective personal equipment used in the care of COVID-19 patients, *Can. J. Anesth.*, **67**(7), pp. 900–901. https://doi.org/10.1007/s12630-020-01648-x.

66. Neupane, B. B., Mainali, S., Sharma, A. and Giri, B. (2019). Optical microscopic study of surface morphology and filtering efficiency of face masks, *PeerJ*, **7**, pp. 1–14. https://doi.org/10.7717/peerj.7142.

67. O'Kelly, E., Pirog, S., Ward, J. and Clarkson, P. J. (2020). Ability of fabric facemasks materials to filter ultrafine particles at coughing velocity - for home made and fabric face mask creation (preprint), Public and Global Health. https://doi.org/https://doi.org/10.1101/2020.04.14.20065375.

68. Offeddu, V., Yung, C. F., Low, M. S. F. and Tam, C. C. (2017). Effectiveness of masks and respirators against respiratory infections in healthcare workers: a systematic review and meta-analysis, *Clin. Infect. Dis.*, **65**(11), pp. 1934–1942. https://doi.org/10.1093/cid/cix681.

69. Phan, L. T., Maita, D., Mortiz, D. C., Weber, R., Fritzen-Pedicini, C., Bleasdale, S. C. and Jones, R. M. (2019). Personal protective equipment doffing practices of healthcare workers, *J. Occup. Environ. Hyg.*, **16**(8), pp. 575–581. https://doi.org/10.1080/15459624.2019.1628350.

70. Potts, M., Prata, N., Walsh, J. and Grossman, A. (2006). Parachute approach to evidence based medicine, *BMJ*, **333**(7570), pp. 701–703. https://doi.org/10.1136/bmj.333.7570.701.

71. Pu, Y., Zheng, J., Chen, F., Long, Y., Wu, H., Li, Q., Yu, S., Wang, X. and Ning, X. (2018). Preparation of polypropylene micro and nanofibers by electrostatic-assisted melt blown and their application, *Polymers*, **10**(9), p. 959. https://doi.org/10.3390/polym10090959.

72. Reid, M. J. A., Saito, S., Nash, D., Scardigli, A., Casalini, C. and Howard, A. A. (2012). Implementation of tuberculosis infection control measures at HIV care and treatment sites in sub-Saharan Africa, *Int. J. Tuberc. Lung Dis.*, **16**(12), pp. 1605–1612. https://doi.org/10.5588/ijtld.12.0033.

73. Reidy, P., Fletcher, T., Shieber, C., Shallcross, J., Towler, H., Ping, M., Kenworthy, L., Silman, N. and Aarons, E. (2017). Personal protective equipment solution for UK military medical personnel working in an Ebola virus disease treatment unit in Sierra Leone, *J. Hosp. Infect.*, **96**(1), pp. 42–48. https://doi.org/10.1016/j.jhin.2017.03.018.

74. Rengasamy, S., Eimer, B., and Shaffer, R. E. (2010). Simple respiratory protection—evaluation of the filtration performance of cloth masks and common fabric materials against 20–1000 nm size particles. *Ann. Occup. Hyg.*, **54**(7), pp. 789–798. https://doi.org/10.1093/annhyg/meq044.

75. Scd, W. W. L. and Sun, Q. (2020). Charged PVDF multilayer nano fiber filter in filtering simulated airborne novel coronavirus (COVID-19) using ambient nano-aerosols, **245**. https://doi.org/10.1016/j.seppur.2020.116887.

76. Hasanah, Setiawati, E. P. and Apriani, L. (2016). Knowledge and intention to use personal protective equipment among health care workers to prevent tuberculosis, *Althea Med. J.*, **3**(1), pp. 120–125.

77. Siegel, J. D., Rhinehart, E., Jackson, M. and Chiarello, L. (2007). 2007 Guideline for isolation precautions: preventing transmission of infectious agents in health care settings, *Am. J. Infect. Control*, **35**(10), pp. S65–S164. https://doi.org/10.1016/j.ajic.2007.10.007.

78. Standard, E. (2014). EN 14683:2014 medical face masks. Requirements and test methods, pp. 1–19. Retrieved from http://www.scpur.com/d/file/content/2018/04/5ae521ad3ab3d.pdf.

79. Sun, Z., Yue, Y., He, W., Jiang, F., Lin, C., David, Y., Pui, H., Liang, Y. and Wang, J. (2020). The antibacterial performance of positively charged and chitosan dipped air filter media, *Build. Environ.*, **180**, p. 107020. https://doi.org/10.1016/j.buildenv.2020.107020.

80. Tabah, A., Ramanan, M., Laupland, K. B., Buetti, N., Cortegiani, A., Mellinghoff, J., Conway, A., Camporota, L., Zappella, N., Elhadi, M., Povoa, P., Amrein, K., Vidal, G., Derde, L., Bassetti, M., Francois, G., Ssi, N. and Waele, J. J. De. (2020). Personal protective equipment and intensive care unit healthcare worker safety in the COVID-19 era (PPE-SAFE): an international survey, *J. Crit. Care*, **59**, pp. 70–75. https://doi.org/10.1016/j.jcrc.2020.06.005.

81. Toyokawa, T., Sunagawa, T., Yahata, Y., Ohyama, T., Kodama, T., Satoh, H., Ueno-Yamamoto, K., Arai, S., Araki, K., Odaira, F., Tsuchihashi, Y., Takahashi, H., Tanaka-Taya, K. and Okabe, N. (2011). Seroprevalence of antibodies to pandemic (H1N1) 2009 influenza virus among health care workers in two general hospitals after first outbreak in Kobe, Japan, *J. Infect.*, **63**(4), pp. 281–287. https://doi.org/10.1016/j.jinf.2011.05.001.

82. Vordos, N., Gkika, D. A., Maliaris, G., Tilkeridis, K. E., Antoniou, A., Bandekas, D. V., and Ch, A. (2020). How 3D printing and social media tackles the PPE shortage during Covid-19 pandemic, *Saf. Sci.*, **130**, p. 104870. https://doi.org/10.1016/j.ssci.2020.104870.

83. Walsh, K. A., Jordan, K., Clyne, B., Rohde, D., Drummond, L., Byrne, P., Ahern, S., Carty, P. G., O'Brien, K. K., O'Murchu, E., O'Neill, M., Smith, S. M., Ryan, M. and Harrington, P. (2020). SARS-CoV-2 detection, viral load and infectivity over the course of an infection, *J. Infect.*, S0163445320304497. https://doi.org/10.1016/j.jinf.2020.06.067.

84. Wells, W. F. (1955). Airborne contagion and air hygiene: an ecological study of droplet infections, *JAMA*, **159**(1), p. 90.

85. Which countries have made wearing face masks compulsory? (2020). Retrieved July 3, 2020, from https://www.aljazeera.com/news/ 2020/04/countries-wearing-face-masks-compulsory-200423094510 867.html.

86. Wise, M. E., De Perio, M., Halpin, J., Jhung, M., Magill, S., Black, S. R., Gerber, S. I., Harriman, K., Rosenberg, J., Borlaug, G., Finelli, L., Olsen, S. J., Swerdlow, D. L. and Kallen, A. J. (2011). Transmission of pandemic (H1N1) 2009 influenza to healthcare personnel in the United States, *Clin. Infect. Dis.*, **52**(1), pp. S198–S204. https://doi.org/10.1093/cid/ciq038.

87. Woon, W., Leung, F. and Sun, Q. (2020). Electrostatic charged nanofiber filter for filtering airborne novel coronavirus (COVID-19) and nano-aerosols, *Sep. Purif. Technol.*, p. 116886. https://doi.org/ 10.1016/j.seppur.2020.116886.

88. World Health Organization. Ebola situation report – 4 November 2015 (2015). Retrieved July 30, 2020, from https://apps.who.int/ iris/bitstream/handle/10665/192654/ebolasitrep_4Nov2015_eng.pdf; jsessionid=C36B39E980B6402ADF4E7E04424876C3?sequence=1.

89. World Health Organization (2020). Rational use of personal protective equipment for coronavirus disease (COVID-19) and considerations during severe shortages (April), pp. 1–28.

90. Xiao, J., Shiu, E. Y. C., Gao, H., Wong, J. Y., Fong, M. W., Ryu, S. and Cowling, B. J. (2020). Nonpharmaceutical measures for pandemic influenza in nonhealthcare settings—personal protective and environmental measures, *Emerging Infect. Dis.*, **26**(5), pp. 967–975. https://doi.org/10.3201/eid2605.190994.

91. Xie, X., Li, Y., Chwang, A. T. Y., Ho, P. L. and Seto, W. H. (2007). How far droplets can move in indoor environments – revisiting the Wells evaporation–falling curve, *Indoor Air*, **17**(3), pp. 211–225. https://doi.org/10.1111/j.1600-0668.2007.00469.x.

92. Zhu, N., Zhang, D., Wang, W., Li, X., Yang, B., Song, J., Zhao, X., Huang, B., Shi, W., Lu, R., Niu, P., Zhan, F., Ma, X., Wang, D., Xu, W., Wu, G., Gao, G. F. and Tan, W. (2020). A novel coronavirus from patients with pneumonia in China, 2019, *N. Engl. J. Med.*, **382**(8), pp. 727–733. https://doi.org/10.1056/NEJMoa2001017.

Chapter 5

Health Service Waste and COVID-19: Monitoring, Risk Assessment, Approaches, and Challenges

Gustavo Marques da Costa[a]
and Chaudhery Mustansar Hussain[b]

[a]*Feevale University, ERS-239, 2755, 93525-075, Novo Hamburgo, Rio Grande do Sul, Brazil*
[b]*Department of Chemistry and Environmental Science, New Jersey Institute of Technology, Newark, NJ 07102, US*
markesdakosta@hotmail.com

The new coronavirus produces the disease classified as COVID-19. The virus is highly transmissible and causes acute respiratory syndrome. This virus can remain on waste surfaces for different lengths of time. Therefore, it is necessary for institutions to take precautions with the storage and disposal of health service waste. The purpose of this article is to present the relationship between health service waste and COVID-19, assessing the risks of such waste, as well as the current challenges in the health area. Waste collection must be carried out by trained collectors using appropriate PPE. Waste management using automated software can control the generation of waste and ensure the environmentally

Living with COVID-19: Economics, Ethics, and Environmental Issues
Edited by Chaudhery Mustansar Hussain and Gustavo Marques da Costa
Copyright © 2022 Jenny Stanford Publishing Pte. Ltd.
ISBN 978-981-4877-78-7 (Hardcover), 978-1-003-16828-7 (eBook)
www.jennystanford.com

correct disposal of this waste. The coronavirus disease (COVID-19) pandemic continues to spread, and its impacts on human health and the economy have intensified day by day. The risk assessment for COVID-19 needs to take into account and document all relevant information available at the time of the assessment. One challenge is to carry out the best practices at home or in health institutions so that there is safe management of waste from health services. Therefore, guidance is essential on the necessary care in relation to health taking into consideration the contracted companies and their servers who will handle the waste contaminated with COVID-19.

5.1 Introduction

At the end of 2019, the world came across a virus, SARS-CoV-2. This new coronavirus produces the disease classified as COVID-19. The virus is highly transmissible and causes an acute respiratory syndrome that ranges from mild cases in about 80% of the patients to very severe cases, with respiratory failure, in 5%–10% of the cases [1]. The World Health Organization (WHO) has declared the outbreak of COVID-19 to be a pandemic, classifying it a high global risk. The epicenter of the outbreak of this pandemic was the city of Wuhan, in China's Hubei Province.

However, today the virus is already present in almost all countries in the world and it is not yet confirmed how the human infection with the virus occurred, one of the hypotheses being that SARS-CoV-2 from an unknown animal may have infected humans [2–4].

In this sense, researchers at the University of Hong Kong showed the first transmission of SARS-CoV-2 from human to human [5]. In addition, the situation is evolving exponentially, with more than 1.8 million confirmed cases of COVID-19 and more than 117,000 deaths as of April 2020 [6]. Around this time, the number of cases in the Americas was around 645 thousand confirmed and 25 thousand deaths [9].

In view of this scenario, what needs to be evaluated is health service waste and coronavirus. According to what is known so far, the new coronavirus can be classified as a biological agent at risk class 3. Following the Risk Classification of Biological Agents, published in 2017, by the Ministry of Health [1], its transmission is of high individual risk and a moderate risk to the community.

The risk depends on the characteristics of the virus, including how well it spreads among people. Among the risks, we have the risk of exposure and in this way, we can assess occupational exposure to waste from health services. Human health risk assessment is a process of gathering and analyzing environmental and health information using specific techniques to support decision-making and the execution, systematically, of actions and articulation within and between sectors for the use and promotion of health, improving the social and living conditions of the populations.

Currently, we know that the coronavirus can remain for different lengths of time on waste surfaces, such as plastic waste (5 days), paper waste (4 to 5 days), glass waste (4 days), aluminum (2 to 8 hours), steel (48 hours), wood (4 days), and surgical gloves (8 hours) [7, 8]. However, some precautions must be considered in relation to health-care waste contaminated or suspected of being contaminated by the new coronavirus, such as the storage of this waste in resistant and disposable bags that are properly closed. Afterward, they must be deposited in suitable waste collectors. In this way, there will be no dissemination of the coronavirus through waste.

In addition, to combat the proliferation of the disease, the WHO suggests measures such as hand hygiene with soap and alcohol gel and the use of tissue to clean secretions. However, with these actions, there will be a significant increase in waste paper towels and packaging to be disposed of, in addition to the increased consumption of water.

Therefore, it is necessary for institutions to take precautions with the storage and disposal of health-care waste and to monitor the amount of contaminated waste being generated. These measures can control risk factors to prevent the spread of the disease and reduce the risk of contamination and contagion of COVID-19. The purpose of this article is to present the relationship between health service waste and COVID-19, assessing the risks of such waste, as well as the current challenges in the health area.

5.2 Sources, Transport, and Environmental Fate of COVID-19

Health service waste is generated by service providers at medical, dental, laboratory, pharmaceutical, and medical teaching and research institutions related to both the human and veterinary populations, who are at potential risk due to the presence of biological materials capable of causing infection, potentially contaminated sharp objects, dangerous chemicals, and even radioactive waste, which require specific care in terms of packaging, transportation, storage, collection, treatment, and final disposal [9].

All waste produced by a patient in isolation at home and by those who provide assistance, if suspected of or confirmed with COVID-19 infection, must be separated, placed in resistant and disposable waste bags, and sealed when the bag is up to two-thirds of its capacity full. The bag must be placed in another clean, resistant, and disposable bag so that the residues are stored in double bags, tightly closed, and identified, so as not to cause problems for the collection worker or the environment. Then, these must be transported to the municipal waste collectors.

The health service provider who monitors the patient's treatment at home can collect the waste generated by the patient for disposal and treatment.

In addition, for mobile prehospital emergency care and interinstitutional transportation of suspected or confirmed cases of infection with the new coronavirus (SARS-CoV-2), the following should be done: improve vehicle ventilation to increase air exchange during transport, always notify the health service in advance where the suspected or confirmed case will be referred, and clean and disinfect all internal surfaces of the vehicle after transport. In this situation, there is more generation of health service waste. The surfaces in question can be disinfected with 70% alcohol, sodium hypochlorite, or another disinfectant indicated for this purpose and following the standard operating procedure defined for cleaning and disinfecting the vehicle and its equipment and performing hand hygiene with alcohol in gel or water and liquid soap.

All waste must be packed in milky-white, waterproof bags made of material resistant to breakage and leakage. The weight limit of the bags must also be respected, that is, they must be replaced when they reach 2/3 of their capacity or at least once every 48 hours. These bags must be identified by the infecting substance symbol, with white background labels, black design, and outlines. During the entire management stage, the bags must remain in sealed packaging containers. The material of these bags must be washable and resistant to breakage, leakage, and tipping. Before disposal, these residues must receive treatment that ensures elimination of the hazardous characteristics of the waste, preservation of natural resources, and compliance with environmental quality and public health standards.

5.3 Monitoring and Analysis Techniques for COVID-19

Health-care waste during patient care, including patients with confirmed COVID-19 infection, is considered to be infectious (infectious, sharp objects and pathological waste) and must be monitored and subsequently analyzed. First, safe collection and disposal in suitable containers must be carried out. In addition, this waste should be treated, preferably at the place where it was generated, and then safely disposed of. If the waste is moved off-site, it is essential to understand where and how it will be treated and disposed of. Waste generated in areas where people wait for medical assistance can be classified as nonhazardous and must be disposed of in black bags and closed completely before collection and disposal by municipal waste services [3].

Waste collection must be carried out by trained collectors using appropriate personal protective equipment (PPE). PPE must be PFF2 masks, gloves, boots, and glasses. After using PPE, it must be sanitized and disinfected. Washing the hands with soap and water and using alcohol gel should be the rule for workers in the internal and external collection.

The Centers for Disease Control and Prevention says that health waste from COVID-19 can be treated in the same way as ordinary health waste. Regulations on how to treat this waste vary by location and may be governed by the state health and environment departments, as well as by the Occupational Health and Safety Administration and the Department of Transport. Generally, to ensure that contaminated waste from health facilities does not cause harm to the public before going to a landfill, it is burned, steam sterilized, or chemically disinfected [10].

Therefore, it is important to increase the capacity to deal with and treat health-care waste. The treatment of such waste should preferably occur through alternative treatment technologies, such as autoclaves or high-temperature burners. In addition, the institution may need to implement systems that help maintain these technologies [6].

Waste management using automated software can control the generation of waste and its destination, create supporting documents, and issue the reports required by environmental agencies. The existing software can assist in the entire waste management process in a company and/or institution. Therefore, it will be more efficient and less costly, lead to better use of time, and ensure more secure data and there will be lesser risk of noncompliance with environmental laws.

Therefore, automation in waste management emerges as a great ally for companies, especially during this coronavirus crisis. Since waste can be monitored in a systematic and organized manner, with automation, a company can increase the agility of processes and the security of information.

The WHO has also proposed a model for the development of environmental health indicators that can be used. The purpose of the model is to provide an instrument for understanding the comprehensive and complex relationships between health and the environment, allowing the analysis of environmental health problems throughout their causal chain.

5.4 COVID-19 in the Socioeconomic Spectrum

In Wuhan, Hubei Province, China, where the new coronavirus emerged, authorities had to build a new medical treatment plant and set up 46 mobile waste treatment facilities. Hospitals generated six times more health waste at the height of the outbreak than before the onset of the crisis, with daily production of health waste reaching 240 tons [10]. Also, there is already an increase in the generation of PPE waste in the United States, according to the Stericycle company, which processed 1.8 billion pounds of health-care waste worldwide in 2018.

With the coronavirus disease (COVID-19) pandemic continuing to spread and its impacts on human health and the economy intensifying day by day, governments have been asked to intensify waste management, including health-care, household, and other hazardous waste, as an urgent and essential public service, to minimize possible secondary impacts on health and the environment [11].

5.5 Risk Assessment Tools for COVID-19

The risk assessment for COVID-19 needs to take into account and document all relevant information available at the time of the assessment. In this way, decision making will be directed and a record of the process will be provided, including which risks and control measures were evaluated, the methods used to evaluate them, why they were considered important, and their order of priority. In this sense, if documented in a consistent manner, the risk assessment may provide a record of the justification for changes throughout the event, including the level of risk assessed, recommended control measures, and key decisions and actions that will be fundamental to consider in the face of the coronavirus pandemic.

The systematic monitoring of public health risks, therefore, aims to assist managers in adopting measures to reduce the number of affected populations, in addition to mitigating the negative social and economic consequences.

5.6 Challenges for COVID-19

If the home health waste with COVID-19 is not adequately collected, it is necessary to request for the competent bodies to do so, requiring that the waste be stored until the next collection. This will ensure that the waste reaches the correct destination and that there is no contamination of the environment.

Another challenge is to carry out the best practices at home or in health institutions so that there is safe management of waste from health services in terms of allocation, responsibility, and sufficient human and material resources to dispose of this waste safely. Therefore, all health-care waste produced during the care of COVID-19 patients must be collected safely in appropriate containers, treated, and safely disposed of, preferably at the location of waste generation [3]. In addition, it is essential that the collectors are made of metal, with a lid and a pedal, and properly identified as "common waste" and "infectious waste."

Yet another challenge is for authorities to clarify the situation, guide the population, and raise awareness among the population and waste pickers about the main diseases in this context and the importance of obtaining this knowledge in order to protect themselves and others.

The population should be aware that people contaminated or suspected of having coronavirus contamination should not leave their waste available in the collectors in front of their homes, as a guideline, but place the waste in two waste bags and make it available only during opening hours. traditional collection.

It is also recommended that a household with a confirmed case of COVID-19 does not deliver recyclable waste to scavengers. This will ensure that these workers are not exposed to risk. However, this information must be passed on to the population so that there is no chain dissemination due to an inappropriate attitude and behavior.

Another challenge and effect of the coronavirus on the environment is the increase in the generation of health and household waste. The population, for being at home in isolation, will consume more and, consequently, generate more waste. However, it is necessary to have selective collection of recyclable waste and have landfills to receive this waste.

5.7 Conclusions and Future Directions

It is important that health service waste with coronavirus is packaged and disposed of in a safe and environmentally correct manner to avoid environmental impacts. The assessment of risk on the basis of systematic documentation provides an important means of identifying where improvements can be made and an evidence base for future risk assessments and responses to events.

There must be adequate waste management to avoid transmission through contact with contaminated waste, considering that COVID-19 has caused various contagions and deaths worldwide. To prevent this disease from reaching more people, it is necessary to adopt containment measures.

Infection prevention and control measures must be implemented by professionals working in health services to prevent or reduce the transmission of microorganisms as much as possible during any health care provided. For this, there is a need for training of the professionals involved. One should not circulate through the health service or even outside the care area for patients with suspected or confirmed infection with the new coronavirus.

Therefore, it is essential to give orientation regarding the necessary care to contracted companies and their servers that will handle the waste contaminated with COVID-19; public servants and urban cleaning workers must undertake technical measures regarding the services provided. Also, it is necessary to remunerate with temporary social assistance waste pickers whose services are interrupted. It is also essential to demand and monitor compliance with what is determined by the competent bodies and to guide the population on how to proceed with contaminated health service waste.

In this context, as many infected people are undergoing treatment at home, the waste generated by them may be infected with the coronavirus and must receive adequate treatment before disposal so that there is no dissemination of the new coronavirus to the population.

References

1. Brasil. Ministerio da Saude. Painel Coronavirus. Available from: <https://covid.saude.gov.br/>, 2020 (accessed on April 2020).
2. Yuen, K., Ye, Z., Fung, S., Chan, C. and Jin, D. (2020). SARS-CoV-2 and COVID-19: the most important research questions, *Cell Biosci.*, **10**, pp. 1–5.
3. World Health Organization (WHO). Available from: <https://apps.who.int/iris/bitstream/handle/10665/331846/WHO-2019-nCoV-IPC_WASH-2020.3-eng.pdf?sequence=1&isAllowed=y>, 2020 (accessed on April 2020).
4. Lam, T. T. Y., Shum, M. H. H., Zhu, H. C., Tong, Y. G., Ni, X. B., Liao, Y. S., Wei, W., Cheung, W. Y. M., Li, W. J., Li, L. F., Leung, G. M., Holmes, E. C., Hu, Y. L. and Guan, Y. (2020). Identification of 2019-nCoV related coronaviruses in Malayan pangolins in Southern China, *BioRxiv*, pp. 1–22.
5. Chan, J. F. W., Yuam, S., Kok, K. H., To, K. K. W., Chu, J., Yang, J., Xing, F., Liu, J., Yip, C. C. Y., Poom, W. E. S., Tspo, H. W., Lo, S. K. F., Chan, K. H., Poon, V. K. M., Chan, W. M., Ip, J. D., Cai, J. P., Cheng, V. C. C., Chen, H., Hui, C. K. M. and Yuen, K. Y. (2020). A familial cluster of pneumonia associated with the 2019 novel cornavirus indicanting person-to-person transmission: a study of a Family cluster, *Lancet*, **395**, pp. 514–523.
6. World Health Organization (WHO). News. OMS: Casos globais de COVID-19 já ultrapassam 1,5 milhão. Available from: <https://news.un.org/pt/story/2020/04/1710132>, 2020 (accessed on April 2020).
7. Kampf, G., Todt, D., Pfaender, S. and Steinamann, E. (2020). Persistence of coronaviruses on inanimate surfaces and their inactivation with biocidal agents, *J. Hosp. Infect.*, **104**, pp. 246–251.
8. PAHO. Organização Pan Americana da Saúde. Available from: <https://www.paho.org/bra/index.php?option=com_content&view=article&id=6101:covid19&Itemid=875>, 2020 (accessed on April 2020).
9. World Health Organization (WHO). Available from: <https://apps.who.int/iris/bitstream/handle/10665/331305/WHO-2019-NcOV-IPC_WASH-2020.1-eng.pdf?sequence=1&isAllowed=y>, 2020 (accessed on April 2020).
10. Theverge. The COVID-19 pandemic is generating tons of medical waste. Available from: <https://www.theverge.com/2020/3/26/21194647/

the-covid-19-pandemic-is-generating-tons-of-medical-waste>, 2020 (accessed on April 2020).

11. Unenvironment. Waste management an essential public service in the fight to beat COVID-19. Available from: <https://www.unenvironment. org/news-and-stories/press-release/waste-management-essential-public-service-fight-beat-covid-19>, 2020 (accessed on April 2020).

Chapter 6

Coronavirus: Exposure and Risk to Workers' Health

Cátia Aguiar Lenz and Michele Antunes

Nursing School, Universidade Feevale, Novo Hamburgo, Rio Grande do Sul, Brazil
lenz@feevale.br, micheleantunes@feevale.br

The infection caused by Sars-CoV-2, also known as coronavirus disease 2019 (COVID-19), can cause diseases ranging from mild to severe. In addition, the virus has a high transmitting impact as it is favored by close and unprotected contact with a patient's secretions or excretions, causing infection mainly, and until now, through salivary droplets. The COVID-19 pandemic context prompted the implementation of measures to prevent and control occupational contamination, especially due to the need for individual and collective protection of professionals who may be infected. Therefore, workers must understand the factors that involve dangers and risks. For this purpose, the theory of multicausality aims to report that the set of risk factors considered in the production of the disease is assessed through the medical clinic and indicators, environmental and biological effects, and exposure. The OHSAS 18001:1999 Standard emphasizes concepts such as danger, it being a source (element) or situation capable of causing losses in terms of damage to health (injuries, illnesses, and damage), damage to

Living with COVID-19: Economics, Ethics, and Environmental Issues
Edited by Chaudhery Mustansar Hussain and Gustavo Marques da Costa
Copyright © 2022 Jenny Stanford Publishing Pte. Ltd.
ISBN 978-981-4877-78-7 (Hardcover), 978-1-003-16828-7 (eBook)
www.jennystanford.com

property (structure), damage to the environment workplace, or a combination of them. Risks are the combination of frequency and probability (of the occurrence of events) associated with the consequences (injury, illness, and damage) of the occurrence of a specific hazardous situation (events that have occurred). It is observed how important it is for professionals to have knowledge about the risks of infection in the work environment, regardless of the area of activity, considering that the virus is present globally. Because of this reality that most countries are facing, it is important to look at the protection of workers in general through the presentation of the protocols for the prevention of COVID-19 among workers exposed to the virus in their work environments. Given the worldwide repercussion and concern on the topic, this chapter will present the protocols used until July 2020, with a focus on recommendations on contagion prevention actions related to occupational exposure of workers in the segments they present.

6.1 Historical Trajectory of Occupational Health

The concern with worker health started in England, through occupational medicine, in the first half of the nineteenth century, with the Industrial Revolution [1]. England established, in 1828, the first service in "occupational health," by hiring doctors to carry out visits in the workplace, to propose measures to protect workers' health and minimize the economic losses resulting from accidents and illness at work. On the other hand, it was a real necessity for the demands of the working class [2].

The English textile industry was a pioneer in hiring a doctor, Dr. Robert Baker, to carry out the activities of the service in occupational health, idealizing the initial practice of occupational medicine as the physician's responsibility to protect the health and physical conditions of the workers. The actions were carried out through visits to the work sectors, verifying the effect of work on people's health, and the influence of causes, aiming at prevention [3].

On the basis of this model, other countries also started to implement occupational health services. To provide medical services to workers, the topic was included in the agenda of the International Labor Organization, created in 1919.

For some time, between the years 1953 and 1959, there were changes in the denomination of "Medical Services at Work," becoming recognized as Recommendation 112 of "Occupational Health Services," after the International Labor Conference in 1958, approved by the National Labor Conference, making the existence of health services in the workplace mandatory [3].

Still, for these authors, Recommendation 112 aims to organize services in the workplace, ensuring the protection of workers against health risks that may result from their work or the conditions in which it is carried out, mainly by contributing to the physical and mental adaptation of workers and, in particular, by ensuring the suitability of work and their placement in workplaces corresponding to their skills, as well as contributing to the establishment and maintenance of the highest possible level of physical and mental well-being of the workers.

In the middle of the twentieth century, after the renovation and reassessment of the concepts of occupational medicine services, worker health became a multiprofessional field. This evolution occurred due to changes in the production processes, in which it was necessary to evaluate the influence of the environment on human health, through the integration of other professionals, expanding the focus of health actions, evaluating hygiene and ergonomics, and thus forming occupational health [4].

On the basis of this model, European social movements subsidized new questions and demands for changes to improve health conditions, the environment, and the quality of life of workers and the population in general. In the 1970s and the 1980s, Brazil suffered the reflexes of these movements, at a time of social reorganization after the end of the military dictatorship and the country's redemocratization, through the Brazilian health reform agenda, in which the concept of worker health took shape in Brazil [4–6].

Occupational health was consolidated in Latin America by revisiting its model, which Arr or to 90 more pragmatic and less ideological, questioning some paradigmatic frameworks that outlined its most intense practice in the early 1980s, helping to determine the health object of the worker as the study of the health-disease process of human groups from the perspective of work in a society that is constantly changing [7].

Following the evolution of the theme, some events that took place in Brazil in 1986, such as the "VIII National Conference on Health" and the "I National Conference on Occupational Health," made it possible to implement the actions by reaffirming to society that health is everyone's right and that workers also had the right to care. Even though before the creation of the Unified Health System (the Sistema Único de Saúde [SUS]), these program proposals occupational health were to consolidate the incorporation to the organization chart and practices of the Ministry of Health [8].

In Brazil, in 1990, occupational health was recognized in the regulation of the performance of the SUS, aiming, among other things, to carry out actions in favor of workers' health, conceptualizing it as follows:

> ... set of activities that, through epidemiological and sanitary surveillance actions, are aimed at promoting and protecting the health of workers, as well as aiming at the recovery and rehabilitation of the health of workers subjected to risks and injuries arising from conditions of work ... [9]

Law 8,080/90 regulates the Federal Constitution of 1988 and is the first organic law of the SUS, providing for the promotion, protection, and recovery of health and the organization and functioning of the corresponding services (Brazil, 1990) [9].

Especially since the 1990s, there have been significant changes in work and jobs, as well as in the economy of organizations. Such changes prioritize the human being as a worker, the quality of life at work, and health and safety in the workplace.

These factors associate the health-work interaction with the importance of increasing productivity, job satisfaction, and significant increase in life expectancy and significant reduction in morbidity and mortality rates, including those related to work activity. In this sense, programs to promote health and safety at work and prevent injuries, occupational diseases, and accidents at work contribute significantly to improving the quality of life of workers.

Teamwork does not presuppose abolishing the specifics of the work, since the technical differences express a wealth of views regarding the work process. Health professionals highlight the need to preserve the specificities of each specialized work, which implies maintaining the related technical differences and adding knowledge to the different daily confrontations in health. Therefore, it expresses a need to make the division of labor more flexible, that is, they carry out interventions specific to their respective areas, but they also carry out common actions, in which knowledge from different fields is integrated.

In practice, however, this effort to unite interdisciplinary knowledge to intervene in the work process encounters deep barriers in terms of compatibility of concepts. It needs to overcome a whole past of where reality is fragmented, reproduced in the training of professionals since graduation, which is reflected in the tendency to maintain islands of knowledge/power and in the fear of the possibility of building bridges with the different areas of knowledge.

The teamwork proposal has been used as a strategy to face the intense process of specialization in the health area. This process tends to vertically deepen knowledge and intervention in individualized aspects of health needs without simultaneously contemplating the articulation of actions and knowledge.

It is observed that in teamwork, the flexibility of the division of labor coexists with the specificities of each professional area but does not go to the extent of proposing another ordering of collective work by reference to the dominant biomedical model, raising the question of inequalities between the different works and the relevance of introducing other approaches to health needs.

Even though the medical professional is responsible for the Occupational Health Medical Control Program (PCMSO), it is known that the occupational nurse is the main manager of the activities related to the program. According to the National Association of Labor Nurses (ANENT), occupational health nurses (ESO), in Brazil, perform services associated with occupational hygiene, safety, and medicine and constitute study teams to protect the health and safety of workers. The responsibilities of the ESO, according to the

ANENT, include varied tasks related to the prevention of diseases and accidents at work and the promotion of health at work [10].

Therefore, occupational nursing has played a decisive role in the planning of the provision of health and safety services in the workplace, where the depth of care and the global character in cost-benefit is perceived. In addition to technical and scientific knowledge, the nurses must have a broad view within the company, which surpasses the horizons of nursing, but without interfering with or exercising another activity not inherent to their functions.

As called by the Ministry of Labor and Employment (MTE), the labor nurse performs activities related to hygiene, medicine, and safety, integrating study teams to preserve health and value of the worker. It is up to this professional to study the safety and dangerous conditions of the company, making observations in the workplace, discussing them with the multidisciplinary team of the Specialized Service in Safety Engineering and Occupational Medicine, and identifying needs for improvements in safety and hygiene of labor [11].

In this sense, the labor nurse must develop and execute plans and programs to protect workers' health, participate in groups that carry out health surveys, carry out surveys of occupational diseases and traumatic injuries, execute and evaluate programs for the prevention of accidents and occupational diseases or nonprofessionals, and develop health education actions, among other activities. The role of the occupational nurse in the prevention of occupational accidents and diseases is also highlighted, according to their competencies and skills [10].

Therefore, the monitoring of nurses in the health/work process in the occupational health environment is clearly seen in the cost-benefit ratio on the one hand, because, for the company, nursing offers health-related monitoring, and offers more security in the working relationship on the other, which in turn, presents better performance. With this activity, it is possible to reduce absenteeism and improve the quality of life of the worker.

Thus, studying the prevention and health promotion practices of workers exposed to COVID-19 suggests evaluating, among other aspects, the exposure of workers to the environment.

6.2 Exposure of Workers to the Environment Labor

It is known that human health may be impaired by contamination associated with the environment, considering infectious diseases, manifesting itself through immediate or long-term events. In view of this, the implementation of occupational contamination prevention and control measures is extremely relevant in health services, especially due to the need for individual protection of professionals who may be infected [12].

From this perspective and in relation to the pandemic context COVID-19, it is important to understand the related factors and occupational exposure in health-care workers.

As per the World Health Organization (WHO), severe acute respiratory syndrome coronavirus 2 (SARS-CoV-2; the corona disease 2019 [COVID-19]) is the seventh identified human coronavirus. It belongs to the subgenus *Sarbecov* of the Coronaviridae family, and it is suspected that bats are its original host [13]. This virus has the ability to cause disease in humans, mainly through the infection of wild animals, which serve as intermediate hosts, feeding on events of recombination and genetic mutation [14].

Given this, and the possible triggers of occupational diseases related to COVID-19, there is a need to understand the field of knowledge called "environmental health." Tambellini and Camara [15] discuss characterization by the relationship between environmental conditions and the standard of living of a population. More broadly, Rouquayrol [16] exposes that diseases occur in a given environment as the result of a multiplicity of political, economic, social, cultural, psychological, genetic, biological, physical, and chemical factors.

Thus, identifying the risks to human health during the process work requires a study of the territory and the target population in order to provide an understanding of the factors involved in the process of health and disease. On the basis of this model, the concept of health and disease focuses on the imbalance between the environmental factors that affect certain societies, which have been modified since the eighteenth and mid-nineteenth centuries, when the ways of life and work gained importance to conceptualize health and occupational diseases [17].

In the context of occupational health, Minayo and Thedim [18] defend the theory of multicausality, which aims to report that the set of risk factors is considered in the production of the disease, assessed through the medical, clinic, and environmental and biological indicators; exposure; and effect.

6.3 Risks and Risk Perception

In the past, there have been many models and forms of expression for "risks." The concepts of risk were built from the relationships that society established following the historical, cultural, and social context of civilizations. In antiquity, there were expressions without consonance, subjective for "risks." Before the Middle Ages, risks were associated with courage and forecasts; in the Middle Ages, risks were associated with religious beliefs and values, natural disasters, hunger, and war; and in modern times, risks are contextualized in the theory of probability.

As a consequence of modernity, for Giddens et al. [19], the concept of risk occurs through historical social construction, representing a mechanism to rationalize and quantify bad luck and to reduce uncertainties. According to this author, risks are a part of social construction; they are not separated from daily activities and decision-making processes.

As per Figueiredo [20], a risk analysis can be done from two perspectives: those cases where the infection has already happened and the cases have been submitted for investigation and those cases that are objects of study with the possibility of the infection happening. In the first case, it is known what the threat is because it has already occurred. In relation to the second, it refers to the potential of risk, in which uncertainty and probability determine the way that societies could follow to avoid risks, which implies thinking about the actions of individuals and institutions.

This change in the concept of risk is a process of maturation and progress of modern science, mainly due to the ability of humans' abstraction to become responsible for their actions and for the construction of their future.

Even so, the discussion is spreading due to the complexity of the topic and the imprecision in distinguishing danger from risk. The terms "dangers" and "risks" have been studied by several areas of knowledge, defining them in their own terms and producing reflections and methods of study. This interdisciplinarity results in more theoretical and other more practical concepts. In this research, some concepts of the social sciences will be approached with the objective of understanding the reasons the subjects are predisposed to risks and dangers, as well as the technical-scientific concepts adopted by Standard OHSAS 18001:1999 [21].

According to Beck [55], the concept of risk is defined as the prediction and control of the future consequences of human actions. And the danger is in the consequences of human actions when people take more chances.

Luhmann [22] establishes a contrast between risks and dangers, both of which have possibilities for future damage, by stating that risk is the result of decisions that undergo an awareness process and dangers are products of external causes. Still, for this author, the risk is based on representations of the dangers linked to human decisions involved in possible damage and the awareness of future losses. In this logic, Luhmann differentiated risks and dangers, but with the same senses of risks.

Sennett [23] points to another reflection and says that a risky attitude can be a defect or a reason for survival; everything depends on the situation of the risk taker. He says that not moving can be a failure, but not progressing will be considered a death in life. The author determines that "risk is proof of character, the important thing [being] to make the effort, seize the opportunity, even when we know that we are condemned to fail" [23].

The main reference, however, when looking to analyze the perception of risk from a cultural and social perspective, is Douglas [24]. The author, when dealing with the theme of risk acceptability [24], starts from the principle of freedom, but, above all, from issues of justice, that is, why do people from certain less developed countries or regions have to receive and accept industries that are highly contaminating and harmful to their lives? It is an analysis that must go beyond economic strategies.

The author [24] also maintains that to consider the perception of risk, laypeople's opinions must also be valued. Experts, from their offices, cannot ignore the social dimension of risks and must always bear in mind public participation in risk resolutions.

Of all forms, Douglas's [24] is crucial when identifying the discourses and social practices of the dangers and uncertainties of people. Their beliefs, values, and all sociocultural relationships are crucial to identifying what they perceive or don't as risk.

Of all these concepts, the most likely is to think that risks are associated with some kind of damage, today or tomorrow, present or future. However, the fundamental characteristic is that these are found in human groups or in all of humanity, in which the characteristics depend on social insertion and its evolution in history. Therefore, in the possibility that in the future, everything can be thought of and conceptualized differently, there is no objective here to identify a single concept for risk but, rather, it is stated that it should be analyzed in an interdisciplinary manner so as not to commit scientific extremism.

To complement the reflections on risks presented by theorists of social sciences and anthropology, the norms brought by organizations and scientific concepts for this topic are presented, aiming at the assessment of the occupational environment, exposure, and risks to human health.

6.4 Occupational Exposure and Human Health Risks

More technically, the OHSAS 18001:1999 Standard [21] emphasizes the concepts for hazards and risks; the first is a source (element) or situation potentially capable of causing losses in terms of damage to health (injuries, illnesses, and damage), damage to property (structure), damage to the workplace environment, or a combination of them. The second is the combination of frequency and probability (of the occurrence of events) associated with the consequences (injury, illness, and damage) of the occurrence of a specific danger situation (events that have occurred).

For Kolluru [25], the risks and dangers are in accordance with the exposure of workers.

The risk is a function of the nature of the danger, accessibility or contact access (potential for exposure), characteristics of the exposed population (receptors), the probability of occurrence, and the magnitude of the exposure and consequences [25].

A hazard is a chemical, biological, or physical agent (including electromagnetic radiation) or a set of conditions that present a source of risk but not the risk itself [25].

Therefore, identifying hazards and assessing risks is of utmost importance for prevention related to occupational exposure of a professional to COVID-19. As such, it is important to mention the Brazilian regulatory standards for the prevention of potential risks and the use of protective equipment, as intense health care of workers does not remove the risks of illness and accidents at work.

These regulatory norms are characterized by NR7 (Occupational Medical Control Program), NR9 (Environmental Risk Prevention Program [PPRA]), and NR4 (Specialized Services in Safety Engineering and Occupational Medicine) and are used as per the assessment of safety and health in the workplace [26].

In this context, the MTE highlights NR7, as it is a rule that regulates the PCMSO, which aims to promote and preserve health and track and make early diagnosis of health problems among workers, aiming at maintaining health, acting at the primary level through medical examinations to monitor workers' health [26].

The implementation of the Occupational Medical Control Program is the responsibility of all companies, regardless of the number of employees or the degree of risk of their activities. It must be implemented on the basis of the health risks of workers, especially those identified in the assessments provided for in the PPRA [26].

To assess the degree of risk of workers' activities, NR9 is mentioned, which is part of the PPRA, which aims to prevent and control occupational exposure to environmental risks, preserving the health and integrity of workers by controlling the occurrence of existing environmental risks or those that may exist in the work environment, such as, chemical, physical, and biological risks, taking into account the protection of the environment and natural resources [26].

The implementation of the PPRA is also the responsibility of all companies, regardless of the number of employees or the degree of risk of their activities. PPRA's actions must be developed in each sector/area of the company, aiming at comprehensiveness and depth according to the characteristics of the risks existing in the workplace and the respective control needs [26].

In addition to NR9 and NR7, there is an assessment of health risks. These are the NR4 and the National Classification of Economic Activities, which highlight the need to assess the degree of risks to the health of employees in the main activities carried out in companies [26].

For preventing these risks, it will be interesting to understand the levels of prevention of risk to workers' health, and Jekel et al. [27] highlight three levels:

- Primary prevention: It interferes with prepathogenic factors, protecting individuals from getting sick through prevention and health promotion.
- Secondary prevention: In this phase, the worker shows signs and symptoms of diseases; the pathogen is installed and active; this level has the objective of preventing sequelae despite not preventing the initial cause of the disease; therefore, it constitutes an early diagnosis, prompt care, and damage limitation.
- Tertiary prevention: It acts in the rehabilitation of the worker, taking measures to avoid the individual's inability to act.

For disease prevention and care of the environment, health surveillance stands out for being understood as a set of actions that provides for the detection of changes in the environment that interfere with human health, organizing the work processes in health, and redefining sanitary practices with the intention of identifying preventive measures and controlling environmental risk factors related to diseases or other health problems [28].

Not only a change in the environment is necessary to protect workers' health and prevent disease but also assessment of workers' exposure to chemical, physical, and biological agents is necessary on use of personal protective equipment (PPE). Thus, some important aspects are briefly highlighted regarding the duties of the worker, the employer, the supplier, and the inspection bodies regarding the use, supply, quality, and inspection of the material used.

The protection risks, safety, and health of workers come under the regulatory standard NR6 – Personal Protective Equipment. According to this standard, PPE is considered to be any device or product for individual use used by the worker and intended to protect against risks that may threaten safety and health at work [26].

It is the duty of the company to provide its employees with PPE, free of charge, appropriate to the risk and in full working order and condition, in the circumstances of lack of protection against the risks of accidents at work or occupational and occupational diseases, when implementing collective protection measures and in emergency situations [26].

The employer's duty is not only to supply PPE but also to purchase the products from suppliers registered with the competent national body in matters of safety and health at work, which will follow manufacturing standards and quality control; acquire the appropriate PPE for the area of activity/sector; require its use; provide guidance on use, safekeeping, and conservation; replace PPE when necessary or lost; take responsibility for periodic maintenance and hygiene; communicate to the MTE about irregularities; and carry out monitoring and inspection of use [26].

In work actions that involve risks to the health and safety of workers, the employer has a duty to provide the PPE. Faced with this reality, employees also have their responsibilities and duties. NR6 provides for employees' responsibilities with regard to PPE and highlights that its use by employees is only for the purpose for which it is intended. The employee is responsible for the custody and conservation of the PPE, in addition to having the responsibility of communicating to the employer any changes that make it unfit for use, complying with the employer's determinations on the proper use of the equipment [26].

It is also necessary to mention the responsibilities of the MTE. The MTE issues, renews, or cancels the manufacturer's registration by the Certificate of Approval, collects PPE samples from the manufacturer or from the supplier company for analysis purposes, and inspects the quality of the PPE [26].

6.5 Severe Acute Respiratory Syndrome Coronavirus 2

The WHO declared in March 2020 the pandemic caused by the new coronavirus, called SARS-CoV-2 and causing the disease called COVID-19, as a public health emergency of international concern. The first reports and evidence on the contamination occurred in Wuhan, China, in late December 2019.

The SARS-CoV-2 virus belongs to the 125 nm SARS-like coronavirus species and is slightly larger than influenza, SARS, and Middle East respiratory syndrome viruses. This new coronavirus shares 79.5% of the genetic sequence with SARS-CoV and 96.2% of homology with a bat coronavirus, suggestive of the *Rhinolophus* virus, indicating it to be a probable offspring [29].

Until now, it is known that transmission is favored by close and unprotected contact with secretions or excretions from an infected person, mainly through salivary droplets, and other body fluids may be involved in the transmission of the new coronavirus, such as unprotected contact. The infected person's blood, feces, vomit, and urine may put another person at risk of the disease, but there is no evidence of this as yet [30, 31].

In addition, scientific evidence has accumulated on the potential for the transmission of COVID-19 by inhaling the virus through aerosol particles, especially over short and medium distances [32]. The incubation period is an average of 5.2 days, with a duration of up to 14 days [33].

Still, according to the Technical Note GVIMS/GGTES/ANVISA N° 07/2020 the Guidelines for the Prevention and Vigil Crone and epidemiológica of infections SARS-CoV-2 (COVID-19) within the Health Services, Brazil's forms presymptomatic, symptomatic, and asymptomatic transmission, as described below [34].

During the "presymptomatic" period, some infected people can transmit the virus, so presymptomatic transmission generally occurs 48 hours before the onset of symptoms. There is evidence that SARS-CoV-2 can be detected 1 to 4 days before the onset of COVID-19 symptoms and, therefore, can be transmitted in the presymptomatic period. Thus, it is possible for people infected with SARS-CoV-2 to transmit the virus before significant symptoms develop. It is important to recognize that presymptomatic transmission also requires the virus to spread via infectious droplets, aerosols (in special situations), or contact with surfaces contaminated by these droplets.

By definition, a symptomatic case of COVID-19 is one where the person has developed signs and symptoms compatible with infection by the SARS-CoV-2 virus. And symptomatic transmission refers to the transmission from a person while he or she is showing symptoms. SARS-CoV-2 is transmitted mainly by symptomatic people, and its presence is higher in the upper respiratory tract (nose and throat) at the beginning of the disease course, mainly from the third day after the onset of symptoms. However, the results of polymerase chain reaction tests can be positive for SARS-CoV-2 from the first signs and symptoms.

An asymptomatic case is characterized by laboratory confirmation of SARS-CoV-2 in an individual who does not develop symptoms. SARS-CoV-2 can also be transmitted by asymptomatic people, so asymptomatic transmission refers to the transmission of the virus from an infected person without a clinical manifestation of COVID-19.

The clinical spectrum of SARS-CoV-2 infection is very broad. The affected patient may have fever, headache, nasal congestion, cough, dyspnea, sore throat, myalgia or arthralgia, fatigue, anorexia, malaise, and/or loss of taste (hypogeusia/ageusia) and smell (hyposmia/anosmia) and the patients may also experience diarrhea, nausea, and vomiting. Bilateral infiltrates in chest imaging exams, increased C-reactive protein, and lymphopenia shown in blood count are the most common changes observed in complementary exams [35, 36].

Older adults and those with associated morbidities, such as chronic respiratory disorders, cardiovascular diseases, diabetes mellitus, and oncological conditions, are at higher risk for infection and may have a more severe and lethal case of the disease than others. Health professionals are recognized as another high-risk group for acquiring this infection [36]. Mortality related to COVID-19 results from a clinical picture with respiratory failure and/or septic shock and/or multiple organ failure [37].

Cases of influenza syndrome (SG), SARS-related hospitalization, and death due to SARS, regardless of hospitalization, that meets the case definition must be notified, as should asymptomatic individuals with laboratory confirmation by molecular or immunological biology of recent infection by COVID-19 [38].

This notification must be made by all health professionals and institutions in the public or private sector, throughout the national territory, in accordance with current national legislation. They must be notified within 24 hours from the initial suspicion of the case or death [38].

When it comes to prevention, one of the guidelines of the WHO is keeping the social distance, that is, people should stay at home as a way to significantly reduce the community transmission of the new coronavirus SARS-CoV-2 [33]. However, this recommendation does not cover individuals who perform essential activities for society, such as health professionals. The presence of these workers in their work environments is necessary to guarantee essential care related to various health problems, such as COVID-19, but it can lead to an increase in unhealthiness due to the high probability of work-related contamination in this new risk condition [39].

6.6 Prevention and Control of the Transmission of SARS-Cov-2 within Health Services: Exposure and Occupational Risk

The health-care worker is characterized as one who works in a health-related environment, whether employed in cleaning, janitorial, or administration services or even as a doctor, a nurse, or a health technician, who are popularly called health professionals. Among the health professionals mentioned, a greater number are in nursing, as they represent approximately 2.2 million people in Brazil, who work in different situations and who are on the front line in providing care irrespective of whether there is a pandemic or not [40].

The pandemic has reinforced the role of nursing and, in the year dedicated to the profession by the World Health Assembly (WHA) with the slogan "Nurses and Midwives, clean care is in your hands!" and through the "Nursing Now" campaign, whose motto is "where there is life there is nursing," the WHA seeks social recognition of nursing's importance in caring for people, family, and environment and collectivity all services of the global health-care network, through its performance, during the pandemic, in terms of surveillance, prevention, control of virus transmission, assistance to the sick, research on COVID-19, and guidelines for the community [41, 42].

It is important and valid to emphasize that health-care workers, seen as a whole, are exposed to several occupational risks from the moment they enter the service [43]. It should be noted that health professionals are recognized as another high-risk group for acquiring this infection [37].

During the pandemic caused by the new coronavirus, the workload of health professionals increased due to the large volume of patients with signs and symptoms of COVID-19 and staff shortages, as in some places, the workers who are part of the group at risk of contracting the disease were removed from work. Overload and extreme fatigue in such situations further challenge the immune system and increase susceptibility to COVID-19 among health-care professionals [44].

A significant portion of cases is related to occupational exposure, as these workers are directly involved in patient care, in addition to insufficient PPE and unsafe working conditions and organizations, which can increase the spread and exposure to the virus [5].

In this context of health-care workers' work practices, occupational risks are present mainly in the hospital environment, as these professionals are routinely exposed to multiple and varied risks related to chemical, physical, biological, psychosocial, and ergonomic agents [45].

Despite the focus of the pandemic being biological risk, a physical risk is also present since the constant use of PPE such as masks and goggles can exert constant pressure on the skin and cause injuries and, additionally, the use of protective aprons and coveralls can limit health-care workers' access to physiological elimination and water and food intake.

The risks related to accidents decrease due to the constant use of protective equipment in times of pandemic. However, accidents cannot be totally eliminated from the work environment and constant attention is essential to avoid and/or minimize injury if an accident does occur [46].

In addition to the occupational risks mentioned and discussed above, there is another one of equal importance, a psychosocial risk, which is related to workers' mental health. Psychosocial risk has a strong incidence in a pandemic period. The fear and uncertainties about pathology and contamination can make workers susceptible to mental illness [46].

At present, some operational service flows have been defined for suspected and confirmed cases and some locations have been chosen to be allocated only to professionals who do not qualify as a risk group. The workers belonging to the risk group, the elderly, and people with chronic illnesses need to be removed or relocated to other sectors of the institution, and those with respiratory symptoms should be removed and tested for COVID-19 [47].

Some institutions of health are making available exclusive areas for the care of infection cases and other patients without flu-like syndromes. The strategy is to provide isolated assistance in these cases and involves an exclusive team for providing assistance [47].

The institutional assistance protocols in these cases are dynamic and are constantly changing. Rapid screening is performed by a nurse, and the case is referred according to the severity of the symptoms and can be seen by the responsible doctor, who provides guidance for isolation and home or hospitalized monitoring, if needed, or even intensive care [47].

In view of the growing number of infected people, including health professionals, it is imperative to ensure strategic action, providing nursing care and assistance to suspected or confirmed patients in COVID-19. In view of the shortage of professionals, the role of students just graduating or in the last year of graduation in certain areas of health is highlighted. It is worth considering safer ways for such students to help in this fight against the pandemic, such as in health promotion and education [48].

Thus, it is essential that competent organizations establish standardized flows for the assistance of these patients, in order to ensure uniform and organized care in all health institutions. The Ministry of Health established service flowcharts on two levels, the nonhospital and the hospital, both further divided into containers or tents and services in nearby areas and/or within health institutions [49].

What stands out for the safe care for both the professional and the user is that the service provider has a duty to provide training to all health professionals to prevent transmission of infectious agents. All health professionals must be trained in the correct and safe use of PPE. The scenario of the COVID-19 pandemic has caused uncertainty among health professionals who work on the front lines to deal with the virus as the epidemiological characteristics of the new coronavirus and its long-term functioning are not yet fully understood [50].

From a manufacturing point of view of actions and joint strategies aimed at effective control against the spread of and in favor of preventive and precautionary care for COVID-19, there must be administrative controls and environmental and engineering methods put in place to mitigate risks. Administrative controls include ensuring the availability of resources for infection prevention and control measures. Environmental and engineering controls are designed to reduce the spread of pathogens by reducing the contamination of surfaces, ensuring the maintenance of social distance among patients and health workers, and identifying areas of isolation for patients confirmed with or suspected of having COVID-19 [51, 52].

It is recommended to adopt standard precautions, reduce contact and droplet transmission among all suspected and confirmed cases of COVID-19, and, in specific situations, use precautions against spread of aerosols. As a practice, health professionals involved in the direct care of patients use surgical gowns, gloves, surgical masks, and eye protection (goggles or face mask). Aprons, N95 masks, PFF2, or equivalent equipment is also used, along with the other PPE. They must not use overlapping gloves, and the goggles/face shield must be exclusive to each professional and undergo cleaning and disinfection immediately after use [51].

Brazilian labor legislation, via the Regulatory Norm for Safety and Health at Work in Health Services (NR32), indicates the obligation of the employer to provide the worker with PPE and collective protection equipment in sufficient quantity, disposable or not, that are necessary for the safe delivery of work tasks. In addition to this, training must be ensured on a continuous basis and the protection of workers guaranteed whenever there is a change in the conditions of exposure to biological agents [51, 52].

In view of the global shortage of PPE for protecting workers and other individuals from exposure to the new coronavirus in health-care settings, it is suggested to minimize the need for PPE and instead use telemedicine to assess suspected cases and use physical barriers, such as glass or plastic panels, to reduce exposure to the virus, and restrict the entry of health-care workers in the rooms where patients infected with COVID-19 are if they are not directly involved in the care of these patients [34].

It is important to manage the assistance scale by appropriately planning and combining activities, the aim being to minimize the number of accesses to the room and the patient [53]. It is recommended that workers who specifically take care of suspected or confirmed cases of COVID-19 do not circulate through other service areas or provide assistance to other patients, and suspected or confirmed cases of COVID-19 should also have limited contact with family. During the transport of these patients, unnecessary manipulations must be avoided to minimize the possibility of contamination of the team and of the materials and equipment [34].

Regarding the monitoring of the health-care professional ex-posed to COVID-19, joint actions involving the sectors of hospital infection control, health and safety, and managers and frontline professionals are essential to minimize the risk of contracting the disease and undesirable health consequences. For this, managers must propose an action plan and flow involving all the conduct associated with contact and infection by the virus [54].

Immediate COVID-19 notification is compulsory by the public and private services, and suspected and/or confirmed cases must be registered in the official system of the Ministry of Health. Contracting COVID-19 by exposure to the virus during the course of work in health services in the private sector justifies social security and labor notification through the Work Accident Communication. As for public servants, it is necessary to observe the laws that govern the professional relationship [34].

The occupational risks that workers take in their daily lives have been exacerbated in view of the level of infectivity of the virus and the consequences of these for the physical and mental health of the whole society. It is essential to know and control the risks to which health-care workers are exposed and to establish strategies for the prevention and minimization of the disease [50].

Therefore, in view of the world scenario experienced during these months of the pandemic, as well as the experiences shared in this period, it is necessary to look at the health preservation of the various professionals who work at the front line and for that, it is extremely important to continue scientific studies, manage epidemiological data, and do systematic evaluations of work environments and the testing of class organs to improve the working conditions of the health professionals.

References

1. Schilling, R. S. F. (1984). More effective prevention in occupational health practice. *Ocupational Medicine*, **34**, pp. 71–79.
2. Moraes, D. S. de L. and Jordao, B. Q. (2002). Degradação De Recursos Hídricos e seus Efeitos sobre a Saúde Humana, *Rev. Saúde Pública* [Online], **36**(3), pp. 370–374. ISSN 0034-8910.
3. Mendes, R. and Dias, E. C. (1999). Saúde dos Trabalhadores. In: Rouqueyrol, M. Z. and Almeida, F. N. (eds). *Epidemiologia & Saúde.* 5ª ed. Rio de Janeiro, Medsi, pp. 431–456.
4. Dias, E. C. and Hoefel, M. G. (2005). O desafio de implementar as ações de saúde do trabalhador no SUS: a estratégia da RENAST. *Ciênc. saúde coletiva* [online], **10**(4), pp. 817–827. ISSN 1413-8123.
5. Berlinguer, G. (1983). *A Saúde nas Fábricas* (Tradução brasileira da 5ª edição italiana - publicada em 1977 - Editada pelo CEBES-HUCITEL, São Paulo).

6. Oddone, I., et al. (1986). *Ambiente De Trabalho: A Luta Dos Trabalhadores Pela Saúde.* 1ª ed. São Paulo, Ucitec.

7. Laurell, A. C. and Noriega, M. (1989). *Processo de produção e saúde: trabalho e desgaste operário.* São Paulo, HUCITEC.

8. Brasil (2018). Ministério da Saúde. Saúde do Trabalhador. História, sujeitos e desafios para o século XXI (Série Fiocruz - Documentos Institucionais. Coleção Saúde, Ambiente e Sustentabilidade) ISBN: 978-85-8110-069-2. Available from: https://portal.fiocruz.br/sites/portal.fiocruz.br/files/documentos/08_saude_trabalhador.pdf (accessed on July 2020).

9. Brasil (1990). Leis, Decretos etc. Lei n. 8.080, de 19 de setembro de 1990. Dispõe sobre as condições para a promoção, proteção e recuperação da saúde, a organização e o funcionamento dos serviços correspondentes e dá outras providências. Available from: <https://www2.camara.leg.br/legin/fed/lei/1990/lei-8080-19-setembro-1990-365093-normaatualizada-pl.pdf (accessed on July 2020).

10. Anent. Associação Nacional de Enfermagem do Trabalho. *Saúde do Trabalhador.* Brasil. Available from: https://anent.org.br/ (accessed on July 2020).

11. Brasil (2020). Ministério de Trabalho e Emprego. Descrição das Funções do Enfermeiro do Trabalho. Available from: http://consulta.mte.gov.br/empregador/cbo/procuracbo/conteudo/tabela3.asp?gg=0&sg=7&gb=1 (accessed on August 2020).

12. Wang, J., Zhou, M. and Liu, F. (2020). Exploring the reasons for healthcare workers infected with novel coronavirus disease 2019 (COVID-19) in China, *J. Hosp. Infect.,* [Internet] [cited 2020 Mar 22]. doi:https://doi.org/10.1016/j.jhin.2020.03.002 (accessed on August 2020).

13. World Health Organization (WHO) (2020). Director-General's opening remarks at the media briefing on COVID-19 - 11 March 2020 [Internet]. Geneva (Switzerland), [cited 2020 Mar 11]. Available from: https://www.who.int/dg/speeches/detail/who-director-general-sopening-remarks-atthe-media-briefing-on-covid-19–11-march-2020 (accessed on August 2020).

14. Tang, C. and Zang, K., et al. (2020). Clinical characteristics of 20,662 patients with COVID-19 in mainland China: a systemic review and meta- analysis. Preprint. *MedRxiv.* doi:https://doi.org/10.1101/2020.04.18.20070565 (23 de abril de 2020).

15. Tambellini, A. T. and Camara, V. M. (1998). A temática saúde e ambiente no processo de desenvolvimento do campo da saúde coletiva: aspectos históricos, conceituais e metodológicos, *Ciênc. saúde coletiva* [online] **3**(2), pp. 47–59. ISSN 1413-8123.

16. Rouquayrol, M. Z. (1983). *Epidemiologia e Saúde*. Editado pela Universidade de Fortaleza — UNIFOR.

17. Roseiro, M. and Takayanagui, A. (2007). Novos Indicadores no Processo Saúde-Doença, *Saúde (Santa Maria)*, **33**(1), pp. 37–42. doi:https://doi.org/10.5902/223658346462.

18. Minayo-Gomez, C. and Thedim-Costa, S. M. da F. (1997). A construção do campo da saúde do trabalhador: percurso e dilemmas, *Cad. Saúde Pública* [Online]). **13**(2), pp. S21–S32. ISSN 0102-311X.

19. Giddens, A., Bauman, Z., Luhmann, N. and Beck, U. (1996). *Las consecuencias perversas de la modernidad*. España, Editorial Anthropos.

20. Figueiredo, J. A. S. (2008). 'Indiferencia o Necessidades Insatisfechas? La Cuestión del Riesgo Tecnológico en "Vale do Rio do Sinos". Tese (Doutorado em Sociologia). Universidad Complutense de Madrid, Espanha.

21. OHSAS 18001 (1999). *Guide to Occupational Health and Safety Management Systems –specification – OHSAS, 18001*, Occupational Health and Safety Assesment Series, Britsh Standards Institution – BSI. London, 16p.

22. Luhmann, N. (1998) *Organización y decisión. Autopiesis, acción y entendimiento comunicativo*. Barcelona, Anthropos/ Universidad Iberoamericana.

23. Sennett, R. (1999). *A Corrosão Do Caráter. Consequências Pessoais do Trabalho no Novo Capitalismo*. (Rio de Janeiro: Record) p. 204.

24. Douglas, M. (1996). *La aceptabilidad del riesgo según las ciencias sociales*, Barcelona. Paidós.

25. Kolluru, R. (1996). Risk assessment and management: a unified approach. In: Kolluru, R. Bartell, S. Pitblado, R. and Stricoff, S. (eds). *Risk Assessment and Management Handbook: For Environmental, Health and Safety Professional*. Boston, Massachusetts, McGraw Hill, Chap. 1, pp. 1.3–1.41.

26. Brasil (2020). Escola Nacional de Inspeção do Trabalho. Normas Regulamentadoras de Segurança e Saúde no Trabalho. Available from: https://enit.trabalho.gov.br/portal/index.php/seguranca-e-saude-no-trabalho/sst-menu/sst-normatizacao/sst-nr-portugues?view=default (accessed on July 2020).

27. Jekel, J. F., Elmore, J. G. and Katz, D. L. (1999). *Epidemiologia, Bioestatística e Medicina Preventiva*. Porto Alegre, Artmed.31. Centers for disease control and prevention (2020). Interim U.S. guidance for risk assessment and public health management of healthcare personnel with potential exposure in a healthcare setting to patients with Coronavirus Disease (COVID-19). Available from: https:// www.cdc.gov/coronavirus/2019-ncov/hcp/guidance-risk-assesment-hcp.html (cited 2020 Mar 22) (accessed on July 2020).

28. Funasa (2020). Fundação Nacional de Saúde. Guia de Vigilância Epidemiológica. Brasília – DF. 1998. Available from: http://portal.saude.gov.br/portal/arquivos/pdf/guia_vig_epi_vol_l.pdf (accessed on August 2020).

29. Gallasch, C. H., et al. (2020). Prevenção relacionada à exposição ocupacional do profissional de saúde no cenário de COVID-19 [Prevention related to the occupational exposure of health professionals workers in the COVID-19 scenario] [Prevención relacionada cone la exposición ocupacional de profesionales de la salud en el scenario COVID-19]. *Revista Enfermagem UERJ*, [S.l.], **28**, p. e49596. ISSN 0104-3552. Available from: <https://www.e-publicacoes.uerj.br/index.php/enfermagemuerj/article/view/49596> (accessed on 21 August 2020).

30. Del Rio, C. and Malani, P. N. (2019). Novel coronavirus: important information for clinicians, *JAMA* [Internet], **323**(11), pp. 1039–1040. doi:https://doi.org/10.1001/jama.2020.1490 (cited 2020 Mar 22).

31. Kim, H. (2020). Outbreak of novel coronavirus (COVID-19): what is the role of radiologists?, *Eur. Radiol.*, **30**, pp. 3266–3267. https://doi.org/10.1007/s00330-020-06748-2 (accessed on July 2020).

32. Morawska, L. and Milton, D. K. (2020). It is time to address airborne transmission of covid-19. Clinical infectious diseases, *Ciaa939*, **70**(1), p. 3. Available from: https://doi.Org/10.1093/Cid/Ciaa939 (accessed on August 2020).

33. Brasil (2020). Ministério da Saúde. Secretaria de Atenção Especializada à Saúde. Departamento de Atenção Hospitalar, Domiciliar e de Urgência. Protocolo de manejo clínico da Covid-19 na Atenção Especializada [recurso eletrônico] / Ministério da Saúde, Secretaria de Atenção Especializada à Saúde, Departamento de Atenção Hospitalar, Domiciliar e de Urgência. – 1. ed. rev. – Brasília: Ministério da Saúde. [48 p.: il. Nota: 1ª edição revisada da obra Protocolo de Manejo Clínico para o Novo Coronavírus (2019-nCoV)]. ISBN 978-85-334-2766-2. World Wide Web: http://bvsms.saude.gov.br/bvs/ publica-

coes/manejo_clinico_covid-19_atencao_ especializada.pdf (accessed on July 2020).

34. Brasil (2020). Agência Nacional de Vigilância Sanitária (ANVISA). Nota Técnica Gvims/Ggtes/Anvisa N° 07/2020 Orientações para Prevenção e Vigilância Epidemiológica das Infecções por Sars-Cov-2 (COVID-19) Dentro dos Serviços de Saúde - 05/08/2020. Available from: http://portal.anvisa.gov.br/documents/33852/271858/NOTA+T%C3%89 CNICA+-GIMS-GGTES-ANVISA+N%C2%BA+07-2020/f487f506-1eba-451f-bccd-06b8f1b0fed6 (accessed on July 2020).

35. Fisher D. and Heymann D. (2020). Q&A: the novel coronavirus outbreak causing COVID-19. *BMC Med* [Internet]. **18**, p. 57. doi:https://doi.org/https://doi.org/10.1186/s12916-020-01533-w (cited 2020 Mar 22).

36. World Health Organization (WHO) (2020). Naming the coronavirus disease (COVID-19) and the virus that causes it, [cited 2020 Mar 20]. Available from: http://who.int/emergencies/diseases/novel-coronavirus-2019/technical-guidance/naming-the-coronavirusdisease-(COVID-2019)-and-the-virus-that-causes-it (accessed on August 2020).

37. Koh, D. (2020). Occupational risks for COVID-19 infection, *Occup. Med.*, **70**(1), p. 3. Available from: https://www.ncbi.nlm.nih.gov/pmc/articles/PMC7107962/ (accessed on August 2020).

38. Brasil (2020). Ministério da Saúde. Definição de caso e notificação [Internet]. Brasília. Available from: https://coronavirus.saude.gov.br/definicao-de-caso-e-notificacao (accessed on August 2020).

39. Brasil (2020). Agência Nacional de Vigilância Sanitária (ANVISA). Orientações para serviços de saúde: medidas de prevenção e controle que devem ser adotadas durante a assistência aos casos suspeitos ou confirmados de infecção pelo novo Coronavírus (SARSCOV-2), [Internet]. Available from: http://portal.anvisa.gov.br/documents/33852/271858/NOTA+T%C3%89CNICA+N%C2%BA+05-2020+GVIMS-GGTES-ANVISA+-+ORIENTA%C3%87%C3%95ES+PARA+A+PREVEN%C3%87%C3%83O+E+O+CONTROLE+DE+INFEC%C3%87%C3%95ES+PELO+NOVO+CORONAV%C3%8DRUS+EM+INSTITUI%C3%87%C3%95ES+DE+LONGA+PERMAN%C3%8ANCIA+PARA+IDOSOS%28ILPI%29/8dcf5820-fe26-49dd-adf9-1cee4e6d3096 (accessed on July 2020).

40. Conselho Federal de Enfermagem (2020). Saúde de Profissionais de Enfermagem é foco em tempos de Covid-19 [Internet]. Brasília: COFEN. Available from: http://www.cofen.gov.br/saude-de-profissionais-de-

enfermagem-e-foco-em-tempos-de-covid-19_78321.html (accessed on July 2020).

41. International Council of Nurses (2020). Nursing now [Internet]. Available from: https://www.icn.ch/what-we-do/campaigns/ nursing-now (accessed on July 2020).

42. World Health Organization (WHO) (2020). What is World Health Day About? [Internet]. Geneva, [acesso em 24 Jul 2020]. Available from: https:// www.who.int/news-room/campaigns/world-health-day/world-health-day-2020 (accessed on August 2020).

43. Cobbold, S., Reindorf, Rel. and Amuzu, E. X. (2017). Occupational health risks of health workers at Komfo Anokye teaching hospital, *Prehospital and Disaster Medicine*, **32**(S1), p. S211. Available from: https://www.cambridge.org/core/journals/prehospital-and-disastermedicine/article/occupational-health-risks-of-health-workers-at-komfo-anokyeteaching-hospital/E133810D457D3 A66620446F8AC420A25 (accessed on August 2020).

44. Zhang, Z., Liu, S., Xiang, M., Li, S., Zhao, D., Huang, C., et al. (2020). Protecting healthcare personnel from 2019-nCoV infection risks: lessons and suggestions, *Front Med.*, Available from: https://www. ncbi.nlm.nih.gov/pmc/articles/PMC7095352/ (accesssed 25/04/ 2020).

45. Arcanjo, R. V. G., Christovam, B. P, Souza, N. V. D de O., Silvino, Z. R. and da Costa, T. F. (2018). Conocimientos y prácticas de los trabajadores de enfermeriía sobre riesgos laborales en la atencioín primaria de salud: un studio de intervencioín, *Enf Global*, **17**(3), pp. 200–237. Available from: http://revistas.um.es/eglobal/article/view/294821 (accessed on July 2020).

46. Bowdle, A. and MunozPrice, S. (2020). Preventing infection of patients and healthcare workers should be the new normal in the era of novel coronavirus epidemics, *Anesthesiology*, Available from: https://anesthesiology.pubs.asahq.org/article.aspx?articleid= 2763452 (accessed on July 2020).

47. Rodrigues, N. H. and Silva, L. G. A. (2020). Gestão da pandemia Coronavírus em um hospital: relato de experiência professional, *J. nurs. health.*, **10**(n.esp.), p. e20104004.

48. Franzoi, M. and Cauduro, F. L. F. (2020). Atuação de estudantes de enfermagem na pandemia de Covid-19. *Cogitare enferm* [Internet]. Available from: http:// dx.doi.org/10.5380/ce.v25i0.73491 (acesso em 30 de agosto 2020).

49. Brasil (2020). Ministério da Saúde. 2ª Etapa Fluxogramas COVID-19 SAES Z [Internet]. Brasília. Available from: https://www.saude.gov.br/images/pdf/2020/marco/20/2-EtapaFluxogramas-COVID-19-SAES-Z.pdf (accessed on July 2020).

50. Silva, J. S., et al. (2020). Reflexiones sobre los riesgos ocupacionales en trabajadores de salud en tiempos pandeímicos por COVID-19, *Revista Cubana de Enfermeriía*, **36**(2), p. e3738.

51. Brasil (2020). Ministério da Saúde. Recomendações de proteção aos trabalhadores dos serviços de saúde no atendimento de COVID-19 e outras síndromes gripais, [Internet]. Available from: https://portalarquivos.saude.gov.br/images/pdf/2020/April/16/01-recomendacoes-de-protecao.pdf (cited 2020 May 07).

52. World Health Organization (WHO) (2020). Rational use of personal protective equipment (PPE) for coronavirus disease (COVID-19), [Internet], [cited 2020 Apr 08]. Available from: https://apps.who.int/iris/bitstream/handle/10665/331498/WHO-2019-nCoV-IPCPPE_use-2020.2-eng.pdf.

53. Janssen, L., Zhuang, Z. and Shaffer, R. (2014). Criteria for the collection of useful respirator performance data in the workplace, [Internet], *J. Occup. Environ. Hyg.*, **11**(4), pp. 218–226. Available from: https://www.ncbi.nlm.nih.gov/pmc/articles/PMC4739800/pdf/nihms753016.pdf (cited 2020 Apr 14).

54. World Health Organization (WHO) (2020). Advice on the use of masks in the community, during home care and in healthcare settings in the context of the novel coronavirus (2019-nCoV) outbreak: interim guidance, Geneva, [Internet]. [cited 2020 Apr 14]. Available from: https://www.who.int/publications-detail/advice-on-the-use-of-masks-in-thecommunity-during-home-care-and-in-healthcare-settings-in-the-context-of-the-novel-coronavirus-(2019-ncov)-outbreak.

55. Beck, U. (2002). *La Sociedad del Riesgo Global* (Madrid, Siglo Veintiuno).

Chapter 7

Ethical Issues in COVID-19

Haide Maria Hupffer,[a] Maicon Artmann,[a] and Wilson Engelmann[b]

[a]*Feevale University, ERS-239, 2755, 93525-075, Novo Hamburgo, Rio Grande do Sul, Brazil*
[b]*UNISINOS, Unisinos Avenue 950, 93525-075, São Leopoldo, Rio Grande do Sul, Brazil*
haide@feevale.br, artmann.maicon@gmail.com, wengelmann@unisinos.br

The greatest health crisis of the twenty-first century exposes the cruel face of socioeconomic inequality promoted by COVID-19, expanding the dramatic differences in access to the benefits of science between rich and poor nations. The study aims to discuss how facing the pandemic requires looking at the ethics of care and solidarity, along with the acceptable limits of risks and damages in drug and vaccine testing, as well as analyzing the supreme power of patent rights so that scientifically validated vaccines are made available free of charge and universally. Responsibility to the other and to the common good are ethical duties that must prevail over economic results.

Living with COVID-19: Economics, Ethics, and Environmental Issues
Edited by Chaudhery Mustansar Hussain and Gustavo Marques da Costa
Copyright © 2022 Jenny Stanford Publishing Pte. Ltd.
ISBN 978-981-4877-78-7 (Hardcover), 978-1-003-16828-7 (eBook)
www.jennystanford.com

7.1 Introduction

The year 2020 is marked by the biggest sanitary and public health crisis in recent history due to a biovirus that does not distinguish between rich and poor and does not choose its victims, putting everyone at risk. However, the advance of COVID-19 across the world shows the most perverse face of social inequality, exposing the wounds of economic, social, and health vulnerability of a significant portion of society.

Even in the face of undoubtedly legitimate purposes, such as the development of vaccines to immunize the human community and the development of efficient drugs to save lives, it is necessary to ask, on one hand, whether it is legitimate to use a group of people as the object of experiments without conducting research on potential risks and, on the other hand, whether the benefits of scientific advancement will be shared equally with society as a whole.

The ethics of care, responsibility, and equitable access to the benefits of science must be non-negotiable values and be at the center of the concerns of scientific practice. Likewise, states and every human being in particular should pay special attention to the spread of fake news and deepfakes that, using artificial intelligence, spread false information according to the interests of the moment, giving rise to a "no man's land," without the faces and names of the creators of these contents. Ethical boundaries and limits are exposed, and it is necessary to reaffirm that human dignity and fundamental human rights must prevail over the exclusive interest of technoscience, research financiers, or society. Strengthening the bonds of mutual responsibility implies and will always imply decisions. COVID-19 demands ethical decisions.

The purpose of this chapter is to present ethical questions imposed by the COVID-19 pandemic, discuss the risks and damages to participants in vaccine and drug research, discuss the effects of fake news in the biggest global health crisis in recent history, and present global strategies that are being discussed to prevent the benefits of science from being unevenly distributed between rich and poor nations on the basis of proposals on compulsory patent licensing and the suspension of patent rights to confront COVID-19.

7.2 Ethical Challenges

The inherent dignity of all members of the human family; equal rights; the right to life; and equitable access to the progress in medicine, science, and technology established in the Universal Declaration of Human Rights (UDHR) and endorsed in the Universal Declaration on Bioethics and Human Rights (UDBHR) are the ethical basis of society and cannot be disrespected in the interests of a state of health emergency. The theme of ethics in science gains centrality in the pandemic, when the sacredness of the human being may be violated by powerful transnational corporations or by the state.

The UDHR, consecrated in 1948, reiterates throughout its text equality among all human beings, the right to equal access to health, and that everyone is equal in dignity and rights. Respect for dignity is an ethical principle that has been universalized for all humanity by the UDHR. When faced with a pandemic situation like COVID-19, the UDHR should seek the foundation for a global ethical agenda that requires cooperation between people and nations, since human good is a common good and positive human rights have a non-negotiable collective dimension.

Signed by 191 countries and published in 2005, the UNESCO UDBHR is considered a milestone in extending the concept of bioethics beyond biomedical issues and highlighting social justice, human dignity, and equality and equity in the distribution of benefits. The UDBHR is based on the following principles: (i) human dignity and human rights, (ii) maximizing benefits and minimizing damage, (iii) respect for the autonomy of individuals in their decisions and individual responsibility, (iv) prior, free, and informed consent of the individual involved on the basis of adequate information, (v) special protection for individuals unable to give consent, (vi) respect for human vulnerability and individual integrity, (vii) respect for the privacy of the individuals involved and the confidentiality of their information, (viii) equality, justice, and equity, (ix) nondiscrimination and nonstigmatization of individuals for any reason that constitutes a violation of human dignity, human rights, and fundamental freedom, (x) respect for cultural diversity and pluralism, (xi) solidarity and collaboration,

(xii) social responsibility and health, (xiii) equitable benefit sharing, (xiv) protection for future generations, and (xv) protection of the environment, the biosphere, and biodiversity. The principles must be understood as complementary and interrelated [16].

The UDBHR, in its objectives, recognizes the "importance of the freedom of scientific research and the benefits resulting from scientific and technological developments," with clear reference that research must be conducted in accordance with the ethical principles set out in the declaration and that "respect human dignity, human rights and fundamental freedoms." In its objectives, it reinforces the promotion of equitable access to results, the "greatest possible dissemination and the rapid sharing of knowledge related to such developments and the sharing of benefits, with particular attention to the needs of developing countries" [16].

It is observed that care and responsibility for human beings are present in all the principles of the UDBHR. That is why, given the demand for a global response to COVID-19, the ethical implications involved in research with drugs and vaccines do not authorize the maximization of risks and side effects for research participants.

In this sense, the saying of Jonas [6] is relevant: "[I]f there is a categorical imperative for humanity, then any suicidal game of chance with that existence is categorically prohibited" and any adventure, "even remotely, must be prevented from the beginning." Once the ethically acceptable limits are exceeded, it is very difficult to go back [6].

Knowledge and how to achieve it is the supreme value of science that at the beginning was guided by its own rules of conduct and by its peers. However, the task of science is increasingly determined by external interests, and when scientific discovery proves feasible, with or without prior consent, the potentials for using this discovery become irresistible in the market for benefit and power, as underlines Jonas [6]. The "experiment" has become a vital element for modern science. In the beginning, the experiment took place on a small scale, and with the advancement of science and market interests, the world became a living laboratory. Jonas points out that experiments on humans and animals are real acts "for whose morality, the interest of knowledge does not issue any blank checks" [6]. For the author, "when the execution of science interpolates with action in the world, it falls within the domain of law, social censorship and moral approval or disapproval" [6]. It is at this moment that internal morality ceases to be territorial, meaning that the same means and ways of acquiring knowledge come to be questioned ethically and modern science faces ethical examination [6].

The current ethical imperative focuses on protecting human beings and researching possible misuse by unknown and unpredictable actors. That is why, the tension between the dissemination of solutions proposed by science that protect human beings and those that threaten them is at the heart of the dilemma of the dual use of research (for good or for evil). In other words, all infectious disease research is also potentially relevant to bioterrorism [11].

The key concern in the governance of science becomes potential risks, which is why it is extremely relevant to weigh the benefits of research with the potential risks and the costs of misuse. This concern starts to demand a new way of governing science. The power of regulation shifts to the scientific community itself by holding scientists and their financiers responsible for the risks of innovation. Thus, the concept of "responsible research and innovation" emerges, based on three principles: (i) opening the debate on what governs the purpose of research and innovation to a broader scope of interested parties, (ii) institutionalizing the regulation of research and innovation, and (iii) redefining the notion of social responsibility in science. Promoting responsible science has become a new ethical imperative to organize the circulation of knowledge in many sectors [11].

Returning to the central theme of the present study, it is easy to reach unanimity about vaccines to face the apocalyptic potential of COVID-19 and its capacity to endanger the human species. The public health system imploded and showed its ills, the world economy was subdued, the income and employment of a significant portion of humanity disappeared, and social disparity widened and showed the cruel face of the misery that can leave more than 100 million people in conditions of extreme poverty. Meanwhile, the epidemic continues at an accelerated pace and raises the question that humanity had never faced before, namely, the equitable sharing of benefits of scientific advances in such a short time and ensuring that there is no discrimination between populations of rich and poor countries.

In the early months of the COVID-19 pandemic, the union of world leaders, scientists, global health actors, private companies, and the pharmaceutical sector showed global solidarity toward the creation of diagnostic tests, vaccines, drugs, personal protective equipment, and life-saving equipment in hospitals. However, as vaccines were tested on humans with promising results, the intense global cooperation underway began to be compromised by richer nations starting to buy all the production of a certain vaccine long before the results of the third phase of vaccine mass testing. What supreme irony!

Countries such as the United States have anticipated the purchase of the entire set of vaccine doses against COVID-19 that pharmaceutical companies Pfizer and BioNTech promise to produce by the end of the year 2020 and much of the production expected for the year 2021, even as the vaccines are still being tested. Certainly, the same will be repeated when the efficiency of drugs for therapeutic situations for those infected with the virus and who have a severe COVID-19 condition is confirmed.

This leads to the following point: one of the main challenges that COVID-19 imposes on humanity is to move toward a more socially beneficial and inclusive ethic. There is a real danger of not being able to cure all patients who need urgent intervention and to carry out mass vaccination in all countries as soon as one vaccine or several vaccines are promising. It is reflected that the economic capacity of rich countries becomes the object of the game in the pharmaceutical market to decide who will be vaccinated and who will receive therapeutic resources when infected by the virus. Choosing for the economic capacity of governments between patients who can be cured and patients who cannot be cured and individuals who receive doses of vaccines violently attacks the central core of the principles that underlie the UDHR, the UDBHR, and the ethical precepts of living in society.

The coronavirus calls for an ethical response from the scientific community and research funders: a commitment to make research results available quickly and openly to ensure that all people can access the results of advances.

7.3 Risk and Harm: Patients and Tests?

Everyone is suffering from the impacts of the pandemic, and the only certainty at this point is that no one is free from the possibility of being next infected and the spread of the virus may come in a second or third wave, expanding the impacts on public health, the economy, science, and the life of each human being.

By the first half of August 2020, the World Health Organization (WHO) had counted 166 vaccines developed for COVID-19 and, of these, more than 30 are in phase 2 of clinical trials (when the study is expanded with hundreds of volunteers) and only 6 are in the last phase of tests (large-scale trials covering thousands of individuals from various countries). It is important to note that before clinical tests with humans, laboratory tests and guinea pigs are required. Therefore, it is only in the third clinical phase that the efficacy and safety are attested from a broader test to observe whether adverse effects occur, what are these effects, and in which group of people they occur more frequently, the aim being to guarantee durability protection and minimize risks. Emergency protocols were used for all three phases. However, it is only after the third phase that the vaccine may or may not be licensed and, consequently, be released for broad development and commercialization.

Neumann-Böhme et al. say that by the end of 2020, humanity will count on the implementation of large-scale vaccination programs to achieve herd immunity and thus protect the lives of the most exposed and most vulnerable people, thereby reducing the health, social, and economic problems of the current crisis. To achieve herd immunity through vaccination, large volumes of vaccines are required and a sufficient proportion of the population must be vaccinated. Consequently, the effectiveness of vaccination programs depends on the availability of vaccines and the individual willingness to be vaccinated. "This willingness could be negatively affected by doubts and worries that exist in the population about the safety and appropriateness of vaccines" [8].

Regarding the individual willingness to be vaccinated, Neumann-Böhme et al. conducted an online survey in April 2020 with a very representative sample of seven European countries (7664 participants). One of the research questions sought to find out how each respondent positioned himself or herself on the willingness to be vaccinated against COVID-19. Of the total participants, 73.9% stated that they would be willing to be vaccinated if a vaccine were available, 18.9% answered that they were not sure, and 7.2% stated that they do not want to be vaccinated. Regarding the interviewees who answered that they were not sure whether they would be vaccinated, the reasons given were (i) there may be potential side effects of a vaccine (55%), (ii) the vaccine may not be safe (15%), (iii) other reasons (30%). In this last category, the most common concern was the fact that the first vaccines are experimental, without any further studies on side effects, and there is the possibility of they not being safe for specific groups, such as people with pre-existing diseases, pregnant women, and allergic people [8].

Neutralizing SARS-CoV-2 (virus responsible for the pandemic) is the object of desire of scientific laboratories, vaccine developers, world leaders, nations, and international organizations such as the United Nations (UN) and the WHO. To disarm the virus, vaccine tests are being applied to humans in record time. On the other hand, public health officials and scientists warn that very quick decisions, without studying the side effects and risks, are very dangerous, because, even though they are rare, these immunological defenders can exacerbate the infection instead of protecting humans against it [7].

Garber [4] highlights hat vaccine developers themselves report that there are numerous concerns that vaccines that generate antibodies to SARS-CoV-2 could bind to the virus without neutralizing it. Furthermore, "the non-neutralizing antibodies could enhance viral entry into cells and viral replication and end up worsening infection instead of offering protection, through the poorly understood phenomenon of ADE." Garber [4] shares in the text the concern of virologist Kevin Gilligan—who advises the company Biologics Consulting on issues of risk and safety, saying: "Because if the gun is jumped, and a vaccine is widely distributed that is disease enhancing, that would be worse than actually not doing any vaccination at all." The author [4] also presents the concern of James Crowe, director of the Vanderbilt Vaccine Center: "[M]ost experts who look at it acknowledge the potential risk but don't see compelling evidence for it in humans right now" [4].

Given the importance of urgently making a vaccine available, Garber [4] brings Glenn's counterpoint from Novavax to the controversy that the risks of early vaccine release for COVID-19 could cause antibody-dependent amplification, or ADE, and facilitate infection, pointing out that for Glenn, the scientific controversy is completely theoretical, given that in laboratory studies, only one phenomenon was observed. Therefore, it is observed that there is no unanimity among vaccine companies. However, the developers themselves are aware that there is a scientific uncertainty about the risks. It is common ground that research groups are discussing the safety of vaccines and that everyone involved wants a safe vaccine against COVID-19. Garber [4] also notes that Gilligan of Biologics Consulting also recognizes that immunization tests are being passed "without the usual amount of preclinical safety/tox data available for guidance." One of the effects of an unsafe vaccine is to make the body even more vulnerable to the virus it is trying to immunize against [4].

As with any vaccine and medication launched on the market, to be ethically acceptable, the risks from them to researchers, research participants, and third parties involved must be minimized and cannot be greater than the social result of the research. In other words, as for any new drug and new immunizer, all scientific protocols must be followed and an acceptable risk must be foreseen, and this cannot be overcome, even in the face of a pandemic such as COVID-19.

On behalf of public interest, "no one, neither the state nor the needy neighbor, has the right" to claim someone's sacrifice for a search for the salvation of others, nor does the common good have the right to invoke the participation of a person in any experiment. A human being "is the most private of the private, its own sphere, not communal, inalienable" [6].

After seven months of the pandemic, there are still many uncertainties about the virus, which is significantly lethal and whose progression and immune response are still largely unknown, which requires a cautious approach and a constant review of risk/benefit assumptions in the application, both for vaccine testing and drug administration. It is important to note that governments are paying attention to new scientific evidence released by the scientific community.

By the first half of August 2020, Brazil had reached the figure of 110,000 victims by COVID-19 and the only hope for Brazil and the rest of the world to contain the advance of the pandemic is related to the rapid development of vaccines to immunize the population and its availability for the entire population.

The expectation on the vaccine gives rise to a gigantic and very economically attractive market for the production of immunizations against COVID-19, which becomes the fuel in the race of vaccine developers and research laboratories to be the first ones with positive results, as it will guarantee high profits. To avoid misunderstandings, it is not claimed that profit is the only interest to developers; it is known that the salvation of the greatest health and socioeconomic crisis lies in the development of safe vaccines.

Under the stress of finding COVID-19 immunization in Brazil, four vaccines are being tested on humans with the approval of the National Health Surveillance Agency: (i) the vaccine developed by the University of Oxford/AstraZeneca, which is going to be produced by Osvaldo Cruz Foundation, (ii) CoronaVac, produced by Chinese Sinovac, in partnership with Butantan Institut and the Government of the State of São Paulo, (iii) the BNT162b1 vaccine, produced by the German biotechnology company BioNTech and the American pharmaceutical company Pfizer, and (iv) the BNT162b2 vaccine, also produced by BioNTech and Pfizer. The State of Paraná has entered into a partnership with Russia to produce the Sputnik V vaccine, which could become the first registered vaccine in the world. The National Health Surveillance Agency is expected to conduct clinical studies in Brazil. Similar operations are spreading across the world.

In a study prepared by Shah et al. [12] on ethics and control of human infections by COVID-19, it is pointed out that to minimize the risks to volunteers and patients undergoing vaccine tests, young people with no background of pre-existing diseases such as diabetes; hypertension; cardiovascular, pulmonary, neurological, or hepatic disease; HIV; cancer; obesity; or tuberculosis should be recruited. All volunteers and patients who participate in the testing must be carefully monitored and followed up n the long term, with special attention to the symptomatic conditions and adverse reactions presented. The authors warn that the regulations and ethical guidelines do not clearly delineate the limits between the risks to the research participants and the social value of the benefit to the community. Recognizing the uncertainty about risks and serious side effects, Shah et al. argue that the scientific community, governments, and society need to pay attention to assess acceptable risk limits in research with patients and volunteers [12].

If, on the one hand, it is necessary to be careful with the risks and side effects that may affect candidates of the vaccines tested for COVID-19, on the other hand, it is imperative to ensure that populations are not excluded from testing [13]. The fear is that rich countries and where the big laboratories are located will test and, if the vaccine proves to be effective, buy all the lots to guarantee the immunization of their population, leaving the rest of the world at the mercy of geopolitical disputes, such as has been exposed before.

An example of this is given by Singh [13] when he draws attention to the exclusion of African populations when the first vaccines were tested. For the author, the ethical imperative to test new candidates for the vaccine requires that citizens of Africa be included, given that their exclusion would represent a waste of precious time in protecting their populations if the tested vaccines prove to be effective in fighting the virus. Singh [13] argues that inclusion in clinical trials is a benefit and a moral right and should be provided for in the research protocols. The inclusion of African populations should be considered because "equity speaks to social justice or fairness" and "notions of solidarity—which requires us to think about how we might stand together to defend the interests of vulnerable groups—and common good—which requires us to share benefits and burdens, and sacrifice for one another, as it will benefit everyone if we do so." Therefore, it would be inconceivable for Africa to be left behind in responding to the COVID-19 pandemic [13].

The WHO points out that the pandemic highlights numerous severe and systemic weaknesses and inequalities, not only in response to the health emergency, but also in relation to hunger and extreme situations of socioeconomic vulnerabilities that are affecting poor populations. The growth of infected people in African countries is on an upward slope and these countries could become, by August 2020, the new epicenter of the coronavirus epidemic. The WHO reported that on July 10, 2020, the African continent had "more deaths from coronavirus in five months than from Ebola in two years." The WHO's efforts are toward a fair allocation of COVID products and that each country should receive a sufficient volume to vaccinate health professionals and social workers at least in the initial phase [19]. In practice, Africa has served as a guinea pig for countless drugs and when an epidemic of this magnitude has set in at the global level, this continent has been forgotten where testing to immunize the population is concerned.

Having an ethical stance toward the African continent also means not exploiting it by using volunteers for testing vaccines and therapeutic trials, as is the case with other research conducted in Africa. The example is given by Teubner [15] in his denunciation of inhumane social practices of access to health. The author mentions that after the African population served as a guinea pig for AIDS medicine research, it did not receive the same treatment in terms of being given advantage of the research results, that is, the availability of medicines for AIDS-infected patients in the African continent was marked by an extremely abusive pricing policy, which prevented access to medication [15].

Not neglecting ethical standards in relation to COVID-19 is to carry out the procedures in accordance with the ethical guidelines and local and international regulations, using the same precautions, whether in Africa, Europe, the Americas, or anywhere on earth. Singh [13] also points out that research to test vaccines for COVID-19 must necessarily involve researchers and local universities, promoting the engagement of stakeholders and the community where the test is applied. COVID-19 shows that all humanity shares a common destiny [13].

In Brazil, Bill 4,023/2020 proposes to amend Law 13,979, of February 6, 2020, and expand section 3 in order to establish guidelines for the distribution of vaccines against COVID-19 to the Brazilian population by states and municipalities. Among the changes, Bill 4,023/2020 proposes the following: (i) to prioritize the most vulnerable people and groups at risk and (ii) to distribute vaccine doses and federal resources to states, the Federal District, and municipalities, which must comply with the technical criteria defined in the bill, such as demographic, epistemological, and health data, including population size, percentage of the population immunized against COVID-19, percentage of vulnerable groups in relation to the total population, percentage of the population already affected by COVID-19, number of cases of deaths and hospitalizations, capacity of the health network, and the potential for the disease to spread in the region [17]. The project seeks to provide transparency to the vaccine distribution process, since there will be great competition between states and municipalities in richer regions to the detriment of the ones that are poor. Adopting an ethical stance requires protecting the vaccines from any geopolitical manipulations of power and more developed economies.

7.4 Fake News

In this section, the intention is to show that in the midst of the pandemic, false information about medicines and home treatments, conspiracy speculations about the origin of the coronavirus, and conspiracy theories of pandemic denial and basic hygiene care are circulating on social networks. The complexity lies in regulating a mass communication tool such as WhatsApp without dangerously approaching censorship related to freedom of expression.

False information shared by social networks that involves public health issues can bring irreversible risks to humans. In a period weakened by the impacts of the pandemic, individual and collective irresponsibility concentrated at the fingertips of those who share and send false information without checking the source is much more impactful and threatening, as it puts people's lives and the public health system at risk. Public interest and accurate information are priceless, and everyone must strive for those. No one is given the free will to create or share content that threatens the well-being of society, based on false research, false diagnoses, and false evidence of drug efficacy.

WhatsApp is a no-man's-land, where the most misleading videos and texts are disseminated, circulating without any censorship and without anyone being able to contain the risks and damages to health. Brazil's leader, who circulates at political events and on digital media with a box of chloroquine medicine, has been going around touting the efficacy of the medication without any scientific proof—an alarming scenario!

The increase in proliferation through social networks and messaging applications in times of pandemic is a matter of concern for the medical area and health agencies, especially when the population is so vulnerable and afraid of being infected or when it shows an attitude of denial against the virus and minimizes the disease. To show the seriousness of this issue, here are some examples of false news items circulating in Brazil: French doctors protested when they discovered that the COVID-19 pandemic is "a scam"; SARS-CoV-2 cannot survive temperatures above 20°C; COVID-19 does not cause pneumonia; COVID-19 causes infertility in males; chloroquine cures 98.7% of the patients with COVID-19; the CRM will remove a doctor who does not prescribe chloroquine; chlorine dioxide can prevent and cure COVID-19; nitazoxanide (Annita) cures COVID-19; ivermectin is the cure for COVID-19; Cuba's success in containing COVID-19 is attributable to chloroquine; Senegal has used chloroquine since the first case and has only five deaths from COVID-19; São Paulo did not register any deaths due to COVID-19 on August 4 and 5 and the actual number of deaths is being hidden from the population; prolonged use of a facial mask causes hypoxia; crowds came out in protest in Berlin against rules to contain COVID-19; the city of Porto Feliz, São Paulo, did not register a death by COVID-19 due to the chloroquine and azithromycin protocol.

The National School of Public Health (ENSP/Fiocruz) conducted research on the main fake news related to COVID-19, received by the Eu Fiscalizo application. The spread of false news puts lives at risk and contributes to "the discrediting of science and global public health institutions, as well as weakening the measures adopted by governments to combat the disease." In a survey carried out between March 17 and April 10, 2020, 65% of the fake news was related to homemade methods to prevent the spread of COVID-19, 20% was related to "homemade methods to cure the disease, 5.7% related to banking scams, 5% mentioned scams on raising money for research institutions and 4.3% referred to the new coronavirus as a political strategy" [10].

As the pandemic progressed, ENSP/Fiocruz researchers conducted a second survey, between April 11 and May 13. It showed that 24.6% of the news claimed that the data released about the pandemic was a political strategy to weaken the government, "10.1% instructed about home methods to prevent the spread of the new coronavirus, 10.1% defended the use of chloroquine and hydroxychloroquine without proof of scientific effectiveness and 7.2% against social detachment." Besides, 5.8% of the news recommended homemade methods for healing, 5.8% said the virus was created in a laboratory, "4.3% declare the use of ivermectin as a cure for the disease, 4.3% are against the use of facial masks and 2.9% defame health professionals" [10].

The population wants to know about the pandemic, and in the information age, there are endless sources of news. There is a constant onslaught of information in real time, and there is an info-epidemic parallel to the COVID-19. Solorzano points out that the question is how to discern real information from fake news and how to interpret information received from different areas of knowledge and information that is difficult for laypeople to understand. Where to look for serious and truthful information about the pandemic is another issue addressed by the author. A large part of the population does not have access to scientific journals, research results, and information from organizations with a scientific reputation [14].

In the examples on fake news, it is observed that the core of the discussion about chloroquine and hydroxychloroquine is in the cure provided by the medicine against COVID-19 and other respiratory syndromes. However, scientific studies indicate that chloroquine and hydroxychloroquine can have serious side effects, such as convulsion, vision disorders, and cardiac arrhythmias and lead to coma [14].

Dissemination through social networks, especially YouTube, Twitter, and WhatsApp, to the general public is extremely dangerous and can put human life at risk, especially when this information is disseminated by recommendations from heads of state, presenting statistical data from research and people supposedly cured and that cannot be proven. Situations such as the health emergency experienced with the coronavirus pandemic require governments to comply with a series of regulations to disseminate data, always supported by science, that is, any information about medicines to respond to the health emergency must be scientifically supported. That is why, no government can carry the banner of a drug or vaccine without being held responsible for any related serious ethical, safety, and moral implications [14].

7.5 Patent Rights for the Common Good: A Necessary Discussion

As previously mentioned, there is a real danger of dependence of poor countries on the manufacture of vaccines and drugs by the companies that hold the patent for these product, of serving as human guinea pigs, and of being at the "end of the line" when the vaccination against coronavirus is approved, compared with the countries that financed the research, thus exposing, in a cruel way, the profound inequality in the distribution of the scientific benefits. Humanity cannot allow human rights to be violated, not even by the smallest minority, because, as Jonas argues, "this undermines the moral basis on which society exists" [6].

The virus does not discriminate, but the fragility in the provision of public services and the structural geopolitical inequalities of much of humanity in equitable access to the benefits of drugs and vaccines expose the wound of profound fragility. There are unacceptable setbacks against human rights and the rule of law. What is required is transparency and accountability from government officials and the entire society [5].

The population density of large urban centers associated with the reflexes of the globalized world facilitated the spread of the coronavirus, requiring for it to respond quickly to science. "It turns out that many of the current technologies that are necessary for actions against the pandemic have some form of intellectual property protection." Seeking the rapid socialization of scientific discoveries, the WHO brought together 194 member states on May 18 and 19, 2020, that culminated in a resolution with public policies on access to scientific innovation to be adopted by member countries, in particular, the guideline for enabling "broad access and open licensing of patents for future vaccines or treatments to combat the COVID-19 pandemic." At the opening of the meeting, the director-general of the WHO, Tedros Adhanom Ghebreyesus, highlighted the importance of making research results available quickly and said that "we need to unleash all the power of science, and offer scalable, usable innovations that benefit everyone, anywhere, at the same time." This statement clearly indicates the WHO's intent to try and avoid traditional market practices in the production and commercialization of medicines and vaccines in relation to the protection of intellectual property and the access of researchers to scientific discoveries [18].

Wachowicz [18] points out that the concern of health authorities is not whether intellectual property exists but how it will be exercised. For the author, in face of the COVID-19 pandemic, the focus of intellectual property management should be the collective interest. In this context, the author indicates that, "in the case of COVID-19, thinking about open licensing aims to eliminate a barrier to the production capacity of the input needed to face the pandemic." Wachowicz [18] notes that the European Union defended at the 73rd World Health Assembly the importance of creating a voluntary pool between researchers and vaccine and drug developers "whereby pharmaceutical companies and producers would forgo the monopoly on the exclusive use of their patents so that other countries with fewer resources could acquire or produce locally." To combat COVID-19, the author predicts that global policy must be focused on democratic access to vaccines and drugs, "that is to say: (i) access with equality, without any type of discrimination; (ii) access with equity in the face of the need of each human being, without distinction; and (iii) access regardless of one's country or region, as it is a global pandemic" [18].

In this context and with the first vaccines released for wide testing, it is observed that even WHO member countries, which initially favored the creation of a new global policy on mandatory licensing and equitable distribution of vaccines, are now changing their positions. The fact is that in July 2020, developed countries that were home to large companies that develop vaccines started a race to buy all vaccine production for their population, long before finishing phase three of clinical studies.

Teubner [15] is right in warning humanity that the issue of human rights is a pressing one, but that there is no prospect of a solution when giant pharmaceutical companies and countries with great capacity for domestic purchasing power and production are involved. One of the problems is related to the domain of patent law for medicines and vaccines, which is why there is a contradiction between the rationality of economic norms and the postulated ethics of equitable distribution of advances in public health. International organizations must be very attentive and act, because in the face of COVID-19, it is not possible to subdue the individual fundamental right of the patient to life, when the integrity of the body and mind is in danger, against the right of property patent of transnational corporations [15].

To face the scenario of monopoly of intellectual property rights (patents) and vaccines by countries with high purchasing power or for specific populations, it is urgent to implement a rigid international policy, based on inclusive ethics, with the aim to prevent the practice of exorbitant prices related to patent, production, and marketing by a single supplier or the collapse in the public health system considering the resources it will have to contribute.

In Brazil, Bill 1.462/20, coauthored by congresspeople from different political parties that aim to change section 71 of Law 9.279, of May 14, 1996, to deal with compulsory license in cases of national emergency arising from a public health emergency declaration of national importance or international importance. In the justification, the coauthors record examples of countries such as Canada, Chile, Israel, Germany, Ecuador, and Colombia that advanced with internal laws and measures aimed at "facilitating access to technologies to face the pandemic, through the concession of compulsory licenses for medicines, vaccines, diagnostic tests and inputs for COVID-19" [2].

The amendment envisaged in Bill 1.462/20 relates to the institution of compulsory licensing of patents, allowing the "patented product or process to be exploited, without authorization by the patent holder, by the State and other companies in order to balance the public interest and the right to property," in cases of national emergency or public interest, when declared by the WHO or an act of the Federal Government. This document provides for the conditions for compulsory license and the remuneration of the patent holder during the pandemic emergency [2]. It must be taken into account that the compulsory license is an exception instrument and it must be very well founded and used with caution.

In Argentina, the Committee for the Defense of Health, Ethics and Human Rights and Service Peace and Justice made a petition to international human rights protection organizations for a free universal vaccine against COVID-19 and that scientifically validated vaccines be considered world heritage. For the authors of the petition, the "vaccine should not have a marketing patent" to facilitate that countries can develop and "distribute it universally and free of charge according to their needs and possibilities based on the transfer of technology" [1].

It is well known that the private sector assumes high investments to develop drugs and vaccines and that it claims that if the project fails and the prognosis is not confirmed, the risk of development falls solely on it. If the patent infringement is authorized, the developer companies position that this attitude may mean a reduction in resources for new research and economic losses running into billions of dollars.

If a large part of the world population is immunized to prevent new waves of the pandemic, billionaire figures are involved and the values for each vaccine can be quite expressive. In the face of a pandemic emergency and if the price charged is not a value considered "fair," both the WHO and the World Trade Organization (WTO) and the World Intellectual Property Organization (WIPO) should adopt firm positions to prevent abuse.

One of the measures that can be adopted, although controversial, is the invocation of section 73 of the Trade-Related Aspects of Intellectual Property Rights (TRIPS) Agreement, which provides for the suspension of the application of patent rights to facilitate the production or import of medicines and vaccines, as described by Oke [9]. A state, under section 73 (b) (iii), can take "any action which it considers necessary for the protection of its essential security interests" during the "time of war or other emergency in international relations." However, Oke [9], in his text, makes it clear that invoking section 73 (b) (iii) is not such a realistic option when it comes to the COVID-19 pandemic as an "emergency in international relations" as some scholars and commentators think. The author points out that situations such as the pandemic must be dealt with in addition to patent law, indicating as a strategy for developing countries to focus on the next steps to increase the capacity of domestic vaccine manufacturing [9].

In a letter sent by Carlos Correa, executive director of the South Center, to Ghebreyesus, director-general of the WHO; Francis Gurry, director-general of the WIPO; and Roberto Azevêdo, director-general of the WTO, with a copy to António Guterres, UN secretary-general, and to Verónica Michelle Bachelet, UN high commissioner for Human Rights, Correa contextualizes the global health and financial crisis caused by COVID-19 and reiterates that access to health must be the main priority and that all efforts must be directed to preserve and protect human life in order to invoke section 73 (b) (iii) of the TRIPS Agreement as a strategy for making vaccines available to everyone [3].

For Correa [3], the use of the exception provided for in section 73 (b) (iii) is sufficient justification to "suspend the enforcement of any intellectual property right (including patents, designs, and trade secrets) that may pose an obstacle to the procurement or local manufacturing of the products and devices necessary to protect their populations." In an effort to justify the use of section 73 of the TRIPS Agreement, Correa argues that it takes courage to face the most unbearable of injustices: to exclude part of humanity from accessing vaccines and medicines [3].

The next steps will be decisive for facing the biggest sanitary and health crisis in recent history, and it is expected that the ethics of caring for others will prevail in the equitable distribution of vaccines and drugs. If the vaccines tested prove to be effective, cost-benefit analysis and purchasing power cannot be the basis for decisions about who will be vaccinated.

The present generation does not want to be marked as the generation of the biovirus that exposed the cruel face of socioeconomic inequality and immoral behavior in the actions of states, vaccine developers, and each individual human being. It is necessary to ensure that no one is left behind. The ethical imperative of care and health for all must be the response of this generation to COVID-19. Humanity is already humiliated by its impotence in the face of the proliferating biovirus and, certainly, it does not want to be embarrassed by policies that discriminate against the benefits of science.

7.6 Conclusion

The ethics of care, responsibility, and equitable access to the benefits of science must be non-negotiable and have to be at the center of the concerns of scientific practice. Likewise, states and, in particular, each human being should pay special attention to the spread of fake news and deepfakes that, using artificial intelligence, spread false information according to the interests of the moment, creating a no-man's-land with faceless and nameless creators.

When it comes to the fair selection of participants for immunization tests against COVID-19, it is necessary to consider a fair distribution of the risks and burdens of the research. The concern that the undue influence of rich countries will enable them to buy all vaccine in production is real and cannot be underestimated. There is a need for universal outrage, including by WHO and UN authorities, against the plight that may be caused by the real risk of discrimination between rich and poor nations to face the pandemic. And this risk is not only between developed and underdeveloped countries, but also within each nation, among people with economic resources and the great mass of socially excluded people.

Ethical boundaries and limits are exposed, and it is necessary to reaffirm that human dignity and fundamental human rights prevail over the exclusive interest of technoscience, research financiers, or society. Strengthening the bonds of mutual responsibility implies and will always imply decisions. COVID-19 demands ethical decisions.

Finally, it is reiterated that the hope on immunization cannot induce movements to make analyses and assessments more flexible. The scientific rigor and the required safety and efficacy data cannot be overlooked. Thus, while immunization is crucial for humanity, reducing the probability of serious and irreversible damage and minimizing risks to participants should be the ethical stance of governments, researchers, and developer companies that are leading research on vaccines.

References

1. Argentina (2020). Committee for the defense of health, ethics and human rights, *Peticion por vacuna universal y gratuita COVID 19*. Available from: <https://docs.google.com/forms/d/e/1FAIpQLSeSYSlmia P0kJwyfl-ZE5jvpHP4ThUxZUVnYVHrJ94jSp6J9g/viewform>.
2. Brazil (2020). Câmara dos Deputados. *Bill 1462/2020*. Available from: <https://www.camara.leg.br/proposicoesWeb/fichadetramitacao? idProposicao=2242787>.
3. Correa, C. (2020). COVID-19 pandemic: access to prevention and treatment is a matter of national and international security, Geneva. Available from: <https://www.southcentre.int/wp-content/uploads/ 2020/04/COVID-19-Open-Letter-REV.pdf>.
4. Garber, K. (2020). Coronavirus vaccine developers wary of errant antibodies, *Nat. Biotechnol.*, Available from: <https://www. nature.com/articles/d41587-020-00016-w?utm_source=other&utm_ medium=other&utm_content=null&utm_campaign=JRCN_2_DD01_CN_ NatureRJ_article_paid_XMOL>.
5. Guterres, A. (2020). We are all in this together: human rights and COVID-19 response and recovery, United Nations. Available from: <https://www.un.org/en/un-coronavirus-communications-team/we- are-all-together-human-rights-and-covid-19-response-and>.
6. Jonas, H. (2013). *Técnica, Medina e Ética: sobre a prática do Princípio Responsabilidade* (Paulus, São Paulo).
7. Landhuis, E. (2020). COVID-19 vaccine developers search for antibodies that 'first do no harm' - biotechs and pharma want to protect patients without triggering immune system havoc, *Sci. Am.*, Available from: <https://www.scientificamerican.com/article/covid-19-vaccine- developers-search-for-antibodies-that-first-do-no-harm1/>.
8. Nuemann-Böhme, S., Varghese, N. E., Sabat, I., Barros, P. P., Brouwer, W., Exel, J., Schreyögg, J. and Stargardt, T. (2020). Once we have it, will we use it? A European survey on willingness to be vaccinated against COVID-19, *Eur. J. Health Econ.*, **1**, p. 3. Available from: <https://www.ncbi.nlm.nih.gov/pmc/articles/PMC7317261/>.
9. Oke, E. K. (2020). Is the national security exception in the TRIPS agreement a realistic option in confronting COVID-19? *Eur. J. Int. Law*, **3**. Available from: <https://www. ejiltalk.org/is-the-national-security- exception-in-the-trips-agreement-a-realistic-option-in-confronting- covid-19/>.

10. Osvaldo Cruz Foundation (2020). Estudo identifica principais fake news relacionadas à COVID-19. Available from: <https://portal.fiocruz. br/noticia/estudo-identifica-principais-fake-news-relacionadas-covid-19>.

11. Rychnovská, D. (2016). Governing dual-use knowledge: from the politics of responsible science to the ethicalization of security, *Security Dialogue*, **47**(4), pp. 310–328. Available from: <https://journals. sagepub.com/doi/10.1177/0967010616658848.

12. Shah, S. K., Miller, F. G., Darton, T. C., Duenas, D., Emerson, C., Lynch, H. F., Jamrozik, E., Jecker, N. S., Kamuya, D., Kapulu, M., Kimmelman, J., Mackay, D., Memoli, M. J., Murphy, S. C., Palacios, R., Richie, T. L., Roestenberg, M., Saxena, A., Saylor, K., Selgelid, M. J., Vaswani, V. and Rid, A. (2020). Ethics of controlled human infection to address COVID-19, *Science*, **368**(6493), pp. 832–834. Available from: <https:// science.sciencemag.org/content/368/6493/832>.

13. Singh, J. A. (2020). The case for why Africa should host COVID-19 candidate vaccine trials, *J. Infect. Dis.*, **222**(30, pp. 351–355. Available from: <https://academic.oup.com/jid/article/222/3/351/5850913>.

14. Solorzano, M. V. (2020). Diplomacia científica: El rol del científico en el manejo de Pandemias, *Rev Bio y Der*, **50**, pp. 255–270. Available from: <https://revistes.ub.edu/index.php/RBD/article/view/31843/32110>.

15. Teubnern, G. (2006). The anonymous matrix: human rights violations by 'private' transnational actors, *Mod. Law Rev.*, **69**(3), pp. 327–346. Available from: <https://www.jstor.org/stable/3699030?seq=1>.

16. United Nations Educational, Scientific and Cultural Organization (2005). Universal declaration on bioethics and human rights, Paris. Available from: <https://www.ufrgs.br/bioetica/undh.htm>.

17. Vieira, A. (2020). Senado federal. *Bill 4. 023*. Available from: <https://legis.senado.leg.br/sdleg-getter/documento?dm= 8871387&ts=1596483052812&disposition=inline>.

18. Wachowicz, M. (2020). Open access to scientific innovation as a means to combat COVID-19, *GRUR Int.*, **8**, pp. 1–2. Available from: <https://academic.oup.com/grurint/advance-article/doi/10.1093/ grurint/ikaa093/5874123>.

19. World Health Organization (2020). *África evita "maior desastre" no combate à pandemia da COVID-19, diz OMS*. Available from: <https://news.un.org/pt/story/2020/07/1719851>.

Chapter 8

Brazil against COVID-19: Analysis from a Typology of Public Policies to Face the Pandemic with Development

Mário Jaime Gomes de Lima[a] and Iara Regina Chaves[b]

[a] Porto Alegre – RGS – RGS – Brasil, Dr. Economia
[b] Porto Alegre – RGS – RGS – Brasil, Dra. Qualidade Ambiental
mariojgl@gmail.com, iara.chavesout@gmail.com

Considered as a field within the study of politics, public policies seek to analyze the behavior of governments in the face of major public issues (Mead, 1995), observed as a set of government actions, to produce specific results and effects (Lynn & Gould, 1980). Public policies can also be defined as a system established between formulation, results, and the environment (Eastone, 1965). For Figueiredo (2009), public policies are related to the existence of market failures, a situation in which the market fails to provide the social optimum desirable to the whole society. Thus, Figueiredo (2009) collaborates in providing a reference for the design, execution, coordination, monitoring, and analysis of public development policies. Therefore, public policies to combat COVID-19 can be considered as policies to promote territorial well-being (Lima & Souza, 2012), based on the market gap in terms of material and immaterial well-being,

Living with COVID-19: Economics, Ethics, and Environmental Issues
Edited by Chaudhery Mustansar Hussain and Gustavo Marques da Costa
Copyright © 2022 Jenny Stanford Publishing Pte. Ltd.
ISBN 978-981-4877-78-7 (Hardcover), 978-1-003-16828-7 (eBook)
www.jennystanford.com

and the idea of "providence state" or "social state," with equity as an intrinsic value of regional development, can be considered a reference paradigm. On the basis of the methodology presented by Figueiredo (2009) and used by Lima and Souza (2012) from a typology of public development policies through market failures and reference paradigms, the study aimed to analyze the types of policies prepared by the Federated States of Brazil to combat COVID-19 and its overflows. The results will make it possible to observe which public policies are being developed by the Brazilian states to face COVID-19 and reduce the negative impacts on the economic development of their territories.

8.1 Public Policies as Instruments of Social Welfare in Territories

8.1.1 The Public Policies

As pioneers in public policy studies, Laswell, Simon, Lindblom, and Eastone made relevant contributions to the compression of this area of the social sciences. Laswell (1936) sought to reconcile the relationship between scientific/academic knowledge and the empirical production of governments, with Simon (1957) observing the existence of a limitation on the rationality of policy makers, while Lindblom (1959) proposed the inclusion of other variables for formulation and analysis of public policies. Finally, Eastone (1965) helped to define that public policies are systems designed by the environment, formulation, and results in which they are designed and implemented.

Thus, it can be considered that public policies study governments on the basis of major public issues (Mead, 1995), observing the production of specific effects (Lynn & Gould, 1980), capable of exercising power and influence in the lives of individuals in society, by acting directly through delegation (Peters, 1986). Public policies also analyze how governments establish what should be done and what should not be done (Dye, 1984), producing questions such as "Who wins what?," "Why?," and "What difference does it make?" (Souza, 2006).

Public policies arise due to a local emergency need, in which the state power seeks subsidies to eradicate or reduce problems in different sectors of society (Secchi, 2013). It is the public policies that appear as a solution to problems of demographic, economic, and social exclusion of specific population groups, environmental, and housing problems, often caused by agglomeration economies (União Européia, 2011).

Poor populations are left out of access to private goods and services, demanding the supply of public goods and services (Rolnik & Klink, 2011). Therefore, state power emerges as the institutional scope capable of providing efficient structures for carrying out decision-making, supported by the construction of public policies (Grostein, 2001).

It is the state power that is responsible for promoting public policies that meet the different demands of society. Consequently, the state power must establish the planning and interaction between governments and society on a permanent basis, fixing and guiding the goals and objectives for the formulation and implementation of public policies (Castro & Oliveira, 2014).

This makes it possible to estimate economic and social problems, providing conditions for the promotion of development (Carvalho et al., 2010), in which public policies are a significant scientific element within political science (Sabatier, 1995). State power carries out political actions in different areas, such as health, public security, work, education, and technology and innovation, involving economic, social, political, and environmental aspects.

Thus, public intentionality is the fundamental element for the establishment and creation of public policies, as a solution to public problems considered relevant to the community (Secchi, 2013). In this dynamic, public policies are seen as the dynamic result of the power struggles arising from the establishment of power relations between economic, political, and social classes, which determine and guide the actions of state power interventions in the economic and social realities of society (Boneti, 2007).

Both the failure and the success of a public policy will depend on the commitment and skills of the stakeholders who are directly involved in its formulation and implementation, becoming defenders of the public policy to be implemented (Sabatier, 1986).

Therefore, it is through the generation of a synergy,[1] with methods and norms, that public policies will guide the actions of public administration, when establishing the relations between public administration and society and between the state and social actors (Evans, 1989).

Therefore, political power is realized through the realization of conflict processes, which are generated during decision-making and which involve the distribution and redistribution of power, as well as the allocation of resources and costs in the provision of public goods and services (Teixeira, 2002). Theoretically and conceptually, public policy theories prove to be multidisciplinary, in an attempt to guide and explain both their nature and their processes, in an attempt to build a general theory, in order to synthesize the different theories of the various social sciences, as in economics (Souza, 2006).

Thus, from the perspective of economic sciences, public policies are associated with market failures (Scarth, 1988). This direct relationship between market failures and public policies exists because the public administration intervenes in seeking to achieve socially optimum conditions that cannot be maximized by private agents (Lima & Souza, 2012).

8.1.2 Public Policies and Development in the COVID-19 Context

Considering the economic aspects at different regional scales, such as the case of Brazilian Federated States, public policies take on a format to achieve regional development by promoting actions of inter-regional equity. From then on, public policies are essentially associated with the existence of regional market failures, in which state power will interfere in the regions to achieve the social optimum, which could not be obtained only by the sum of decisions by private actors (Lima & Souza, 2012).

In this context, the existence of a health crisis, such as the incidence of the pandemic of COVID-19, resulting from the new coronavirus, is a market failure that requires the existence of

---

[1] For Evans (1989), synergy involves the relationships between governments and groups of engaged citizens that reinforce each other.

public policies that can guarantee not only the establishment of health conditions for protecting the territories but also the establishment of public policies that also guarantee the survival of the entrepreneurial capacity and generation of development in the territories. Because COVID-19 does not have a vaccine or a proven safe and efficient treatment, it requires the presence of state power to reduce the negative impacts of its effects, both on the population's health and on the economy.

Understanding the transversalization of public policies, such as the actions that integrate public administration in its different spheres, by ensuring that the policies evolve according to a multivariate behavior, it becomes possible to establish a reference for the construction, systematization, and critical analysis of public policies, built centrally, regionally, and locally (Figueiredo, 2009). On the basis of this, Figueiredo (2009) created a typology of public development policies based on market failures.

From an institutional framework point of view, public policies can be systematized according to the market failures that justify their existence, with the paradigms of the regional economy formatting an analysis framework (Figueiredo, 2009).

In this sense, different types of public policies emerge, according to the existing market failures in the regions. Table 8.1 shows two types of public policies relevant to the maintenance and resumption of the economic development of the territories before COVID-19:

> Public policies for mobilizing and valuing endogenous capital are aimed at comparative advantages and the external valuation of endogenous resources that must be mobilized and valued, such as the protection, mobilization, and valuation of workers and local enterprises. This type of policy considers that everything can be imported, with the exception of the development process (Lima & Souza, 2012).

Public policies for mobilizing and valuing the externalities of business competitiveness, nevertheless, seek to influence the external environment of companies. In addition to being directed to the productive infrastructure, they consider the regions as a matrix for the generation, learning, and accumulation of business knowledge. Hence, the actions promoted by these policies must

Table 8.1 Types of public policies according to market failures and reference paradigms

Public policy typologies	Objectives and nature of the supplementary role in relation to the market	Paradigm reference	Description
Public policies for mobilizing and valuing endogenous capital	Removing vicious circles and blocking resource mobilization and enhancement, enabling externalities of demand	Sustained development and a bottom-up approach—"endogenous development"	Policies that act in the institutional field, seeking to integrate the development process
Public policies for promoting and enhancing the externalities of business competitiveness	Intervening in the external environment of the competitiveness of companies	Agglomeration economy and implicit knowledge; the (innovative) environment as an intangible economic asset; models of endogenous growth and externalities	Public policies grounded in and organized on the basis of the concept of external impacts (externalities) on territorial and regional problems

Source: Created as per Figueiredo (2009) and Lima and Souza (2013).

be oriented toward technological innovation and the formation of regional clusters (Lima & Souza, 2012).

The states that belong to the Federative Republic of Brazil have taken several actions to prevent the pandemic from advancing and reduce its negative impacts on the economy. It is important to observe the public policies that these states are implementing to guarantee a minimum social survival situation for society inserted in their territories, considering the need to protect workers and productive enterprises that guarantee regional development, as well as to enable the circumstances for economic resumption of productive activities in the post-pandemic days.

8.2 Policies of Federated States to Combat the Negative Effects of COVID-19 on Development

8.2.1 Contextualization of COVID-19 in Brazil

In 2020, the world economy and the Brazilian economy showed a resumption of economic growth. The Brazilian economy had been maintaining a uniform level of growth since 2017, after successive negative growths in the years 2015 and 2016. The expectation was that in 2020, Brazil could finally reestablish the resumption of the economic growth cycle.

In March 2020, it was observed that the resumption would not occur as expected, as a result of the arrival of COVID-19 in the country. It being a disease without a vaccine and safe and efficient treatment, the approach of combating the pandemic adopted in Brazil was of social distancing, in accordance with scientific studies and the World Health Organization recommendation. This significantly impacted the economy in terms of demand and supply, causing the closing of companies and an increase in unemployment.

The International Monetary Fund (IMF), as a result, presented a pessimistic projection for the Brazilian economy for the year 2020, with an expected resumption in the economy only from 2021. According to the IMF (2020), the Brazilian economy will behave as follows:

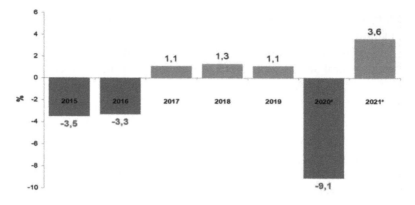

Figure 8.1 Brazil's GDP behavior (2015–2021). Sourced from the IMF, 2020. The asterisk (*) signifies a forecast of the economy.

The impact of COVID-19 on the Brazilian economy has significantly slowed the recovery of the national economy. The IMF (2020) expects the gross domestic product (GDP) to decline by 9.1% for the year 2020, with a gradual recovery starting in 2021, with a GDP of 3.6%. This will affect the markets and the Brazilian private economy, as well as the public accounts.

The Federative Republic of Brazil, through its Federal Constitution, organizes the political-administrative organization of the Brazilian state in three areas for the realization of public policies: union, states, and municipalities (Constituição Federal, 1988). With this format, the governance of public policies in Brazil can be classified as Type I multilevel governance (MLG).[2]

This type of governance is inspired by federalism,[3] with a limited number of jurisdictions that combine multiple functions, bringing together a variety of public policy responsibilities. Having their

---

[2]"... it is a desirable approach to government decision-making processes as it promotes a greater emphasis on the cooperative rather than competitive processes in intergovernmental relations. The MLG is also desirable due to the horizontal expansion of public decision making to include non-governmental and civil-society actors and its vertical expansion, to encompass both local and supranational levels of government" (Lima, 2018, p. 67).

[3]Although federalism is influenced by Type I governance systems, these systems are not limited by this form of governance, not even by the nation-state (Stein & Turkewitsch, 2008).

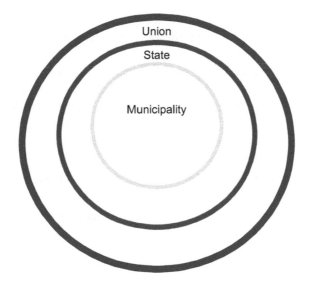

Figure 8.2   Type I multilevel governance. Sourced from Lima (2018).

own representative institutions and their own judiciary, they act as general-purpose governance (Best, 2011).

Type I governance acts as a self-government, with provision for allocating competencies to the different levels of government, with appropriate instruments for carrying out public policies. Usually, the competencies for the execution of public policies are shared or overlap. However, they are characterized by the clear division of hierarchical power (Hooghe & Marks, 2003). The configuration of Type 1 MLG can be seen in Fig. 8.2.

From the aforementioned considerations, the study will observe, within the Brazilian Federated States, (i) public policies for mobilizing and enhancing the externalities of business competitiveness and (ii) public policies for mobilizing and valuing the externalities of business competitiveness.

It is important to observe these public policies within the Brazilian Federated States during the pandemic due to the criticism Brazilian federalism is facing. At the current juncture, with the existence of transversal public policies, with shared management in many areas, the union has avoided investment responsibility (Abrucio & Franzese, 2007).

This increases the dependence of states on the union. Such dependence could only be minimized through fiscal decentralization (Soares & Machado, 2018).

Consequently, the union merely transfers functions, without the necessary financial resources, for the Brazilian Federated States to carry out different policies in a situation of great indebtedness and low financial availability. Therefore, it is important to observe what actions these states are taking to confront the situation created by COVID-19, as these subnational entities have been organizing to confront the pandemic in the current federative conjuncture.

8.2.2 Public Policies Developed by Brazilian Federated States to Fight the Effects of COVID-19

8.2.2.1 COVID-19 in Brazil

Brazil has 26 Federated States and a Federal District (Distrito Federal), where the federal capital, Brasília, is located. The most populous state is São Paulo, with approximately 46 million inhabitants. The least populous is the State of Roraima, with about 500,000 inhabitants.

All Brazilian Federated States are showing, to a lesser or greater degree, COVID-19 presence, and the population size is not always related to the level of mortality. In addition to having the largest population, São Paulo has been presenting the highest number of cases of COVID-19 (697,530 as), together with the number of deaths (26,780). The state with the lowest number of cases so far has been the State of Acre (22,516), while the State of Tocantins has the lowest number of deaths (506). The data are as of August 2020.

In regard to mortality per hundred thousand inhabitants, Roraima is the state with the highest number (93.8 per hundred thousand inhabitants), while the state with the smallest number is Minas Gerais (19.1 per hundred thousand inhabitants). Table 8.2 shows the Brazilian Federated States, with their respective populations, and the number of infected and deaths due to COVID-19 as of August 2020.

Among the 26 states and the Federal District, only 10 are below the mortality per hundred thousand inhabitants of the Brazilian

Table 8.2 Federated States, population, and cases of COVID-19

	States	Number of inhabitants	Number of COVID-19 cases	Number of deaths caused by COVID-19	Mortality/ 100,000 inhabitants
1	Acre	881,935	22,516	576	65.3
2	Alagoas	3,337,357	72,076	1,742	52.2
3	Amapá	845,731	39,431	613	72.5
4	Amazonas	4,144,597	111,241	3,463	83.6
5	Bahia	14,873,064	214,379	4,338	29.2
6	Ceará	9,132,078	197,381	8,129	89
7	Distrito Federal*	3,015,268	135,014	1,958	64.9
8	Espírito Santo	4,018,650	98,765	2,864	71.3
9	Goiás	7,018,354	100,938	2,286	32.6
10	Maranhão	7,075,181	136,280	3,253	46
11	Mato Grosso	3,484,466	72,761	2,319	66.6
12	Mato Grosso do Sul	2,778,986	36,542	598	21.5
13	Minas Gerais	21,168,791	171,514	4,044	19.1
14	Pará	8,602,865	177,010	5,932	69
15	Paraíba	4,018,127	95,588	2,138	53.2
16	Paraná	11,433,957	103,771	2,665	23.3
17	Pernambuco	9,557,071	111,773	7,156	74.9
18	Piauí	3,273,227	65,638	1,594	48.7
19	Rio de Janeiro	17,264,943	190,614	14,526	84.1
20	Rio Grande do Norte	3,506,853	57,660	2,062	58.8
21	Rio Grande do Sul	11,377,239	97,445	2,647	23.3
22	Rondônia	1,777,225	47,652	1,012	56.9
23	Roraima	605,761	39,397	568	93.8
24	Santa Catarina	7,164,788	120,001	1,767	24.7
25	São Paulo	45,919,049	697,530	26,780	58.3
26	Sergipe	2,298,696	67,701	1,696	73.8
27	Tocantins	1,572,866	36,478	506	32.2
	Total Brazil	**210,147,125**	**3,317,096**	**107,232**	**51**

Source: Brazilian Institute of Geography and Statistics (2020)/Painel Coronavírus (2020). The data are as on August 15, 2020.
*Federal District

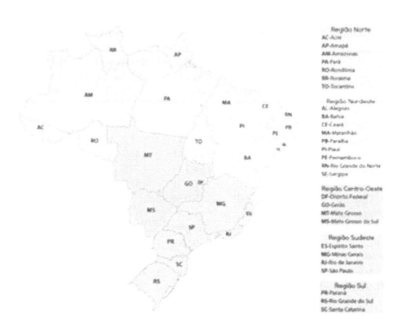

Figure 8.3 Brazil political-administrative division (Federated States). Sourced from Info Escola (2020).

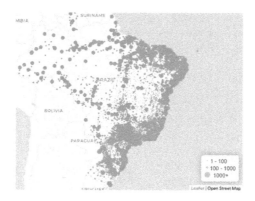

Figure 8.4 Brazil COVID-19 cases. Sourced from Painel Coronavírus (2020).

average (51 per hundred thousand inhabitants). The figures below show the political and administrative division of Brazil by the Federated States and their respective numbers of COVID-19 cases and the level of existing deaths.

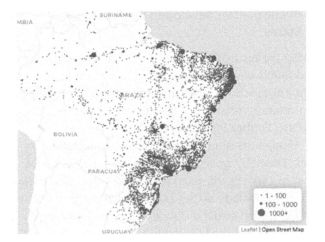

Figure 8.5   Brazil: Deaths. Sourced from Painel Coronavírus (2020).

The incidence of cases resulted in several efforts by the Brazilian public administration, particularly in regard to reducing the level of contagion. The strategy adopted by the states and municipalities was the social distancing, while the union was more concerned with maintaining economic activity, expanding credit for companies, and enabling a minimum social income for disadvantaged people and self-employed professionals during the pandemic.

Under pressure by the National Congress, the union carried out several on-lending programs for the losses of revenue from municipalities and states.[4] Thus, it remained for municipalities and states to focus on actions aimed at controlling the transmission and contagion of COVID-19, as well as actions aimed at assisting the productive activity located in their territories.

Therefore, the public policies developed by the Federated States and the Federal District, are analyzed. All policies created in this period to combat COVID-19 and its effects on the economy and society will be understood.

---

[4] This was because only the Federal Government has the capacity to raise funds from third parties (indebtedness), since the enactment of the Fiscal Responsibility Law (Federal Complementary Law N° 101/2000).

8.2.2.2 Public policies developed by the Brazilian Federated States

Considering the incidence of the COVID-19 pandemic, the Brazilian Federated States have developed actions to combat and control the pandemic. These actions focus on monitoring and security protocols, while maintaining relations with the municipalities, for decision-making (Patri Política Públicas, 2020).

Even though in some states conflicts occurred as a result of actions taken by governors, there was convergence in many measures. In this regard, one of the Federated States that draws attention is Rio Grande do Sul (southern Brazil), which adopted a model of controlled social distance as per the contagious situation of the territories and the hospital infrastructure, identified by flags, from the mildest restriction (yellow flag) to the most radical one (black flag), maintaining constant dialogue with the federation of municipalities in that state (Patri Política Públicas, 2020).

The resulting (i) public policies for mobilizing and valuing endogenous capital and (ii) public policies for mobilizing and valuing the externalities of business competitiveness, which the governments of the Federated States have implemented to combat the effects of COVID-19 on development, can be seen in Table 8.3.

From Table 8.3, it can be observed that many Federated States have not taken actions aimed at the valorization of endogenous capital and the externalities of business competitiveness, such as the States of Acre, Alagoas, Mato Grosso do Sul, Paraíba, Pernambuco, Piauí, Rio Grande do Norte, Rio Grande do Sul, Roraima, São Paulo, Sergipe, and Tocantins. Thus, almost 50% of the Federated States (46.2%) did not elaborate public policies through exclusive laws to face COVID-19 and its impacts on economic development.

This situation can be explained by the existence of previous public policies for regional development in these states, enabling the possibility to direct the efforts of these policies through executive decrees. Therefore, these states made efforts to directly combat the spread of contagion from COVID-19 (Estaduais, 2020).

Table 8.3 Public policies created by the Federated States for mobilizing and valuing (i) endogenous capital and (ii) externalities of business competitiveness

States	Public policies for mobilizing and valuing endogenous capital	Public policies for mobilizing and valuing the externalities of business competitiveness
Acre	– X –	– X –
Alagoas	– X –	– X –
Amapá	LAW N° 2.501, DE 30 DE ABRIL DE 2020: Instituted an emergency financial assistance, called Emergency Citizen Income, in favor of families in social vulnerability, destined to the acquisition of a "basic-needs grocery package," made up of food products and personal hygiene and cleaning materials, as a form of assistance given during the condition of public and economic calamity caused by the COVID-19 pandemic.	– X –
Amazonas	LAW N° 5.161, DE 02 DE ABRIL DE 2020: Authorized the purchase of inputs by the public administration, using those accredited by the School Lunch Regionalization Program and producers registered at the fairs of the Amazonas Sustainable Development Agency, to handle the needs arising from the COVID-19 pandemic.	– X –
Bahia	LAW N° 14.264, DE 15 DE MAIO 2020: Instituted financial assistance in favor of individuals infected with the new coronavirus who accepted being hosted in the Reception and Clinical Monitoring Centers of the State of Bahia.	– X –

(Contd.)

Table 8.3 *(Contd.)*

States	Public policies for mobilizing and valuing endogenous capital	Public policies for mobilizing and valuing the externalities of business competitiveness
Ceará	LAW N° 17.243, 21 DE JULHO DE 2020: Assured the consumer, in the State of Ceará that the contracted event package could be rescheduled due to the COVID-19 disease, caused by the new coronavirus. LAW N° 17.223, 12 DE JUNHO DE 2020: Guaranteed students the replacement of suspended classes by making it obligatory for fitness centers and similar establishments not performing their activities remotely to extend the final date of the promotional plans acquired and paid before the establishment of the social isolation determined by the contingency plan to combat the COVID-19 pandemic. COMPLEMENTARY LAW N° 213, 27 DE MARÇO DE 2020: Rendered the provisions of this law inapplicable, exceptionally, during the health emergency situation decreed in an act of the Executive Branch due to the new Coronavirus (COVID-19), to the procedure for entering into partnership for cultural projects developed by individuals within the State Culture System (Siec).	– X –

Distrito Federal*	LAW N° 6.629, DE 7 DE JULHO DE 2020: Instituted the Emergency Business Credit Program of the Federal District (PROCRED-DF) to face the economic effects of the public health emergency of international importance resulting from the COVID-19 pandemic and created its Guarantee Fund (FG/PROCRED-DF). LAW N° 6.621, DE 11 DE JUNHO DE 2020: Granted financial assistance to the owners of buses and minibuses or other vehicles intended for public school and tourism transportation that provide services upon concession or permission from the government and that were appropriately registered on January 31, 2020.
Espírito Santo	LAW N° 11.125, DE 06 DE ABRIL DE 2020: Authorized the state to associate with the private fund to be created by the Development Bank of Espírito Santo (BANDES) in order to directly guarantee the risk in credit operations for individual microentrepreneurs, microenterprises, and small companies; family farming cooperatives in Espírito Santo, unions of family farmers, and associations of small family farmers; and associations and colonies of fishermen, shellfish-gatherers, and the like as well as associations of professional artisanal fishermen and aquaculture farmers.

(Contd.)

Table 8.3 *(Contd.)*

States	Public policies for mobilizing and valuing endogenous capital	Public policies for mobilizing and valuing the externalities of business competitiveness
Goiás	LAW N° 20.773, DE 08 DE MAIO DE 2020: Instituted the Extraordinary Environmental Licensing Regime (REL) as a measure to face the extreme economic situation in the State of Goiás caused by the decree of a state of public calamity resulting from the human infection with the new coronavirus (COVID-19). LAW N° 20.793, DE 09 DE JUNHO DE 2020: Provided for the creation of a revolving fund within the State Secretariat for Development and Innovation (SEDI).	LAW N° 20.793, DE 09 DE JUNHO DE 2020: Provided for the creation of a revolving fund within the SEDI.
Maranhão	LAW N° 11.256, DE 27 DE ABRIL DE 2020: Exempted from the payment of the tax on transactions related to the Circulation of Goods and Provision of Interstate and Intermunicipal Transport and Communication Services until July 31, 2020; internal, interstate, and import operations; as well as the corresponding transport services practiced by individuals and legal entities, taxpayers or not, carried out with the equipment, supplies, and goods destined to combat, prevent, and cope with the contingency of COVID-19, an infectious disease caused by the new coronavirus (SARS-CoV-2).	LAW N° 11.256, DE 27 DE ABRIL DE 2020: Exempted from the payment of the tax on transactions related to the Circulation of Goods and Provision of Interstate and Intermunicipal Transport and Communication Services until July 31, 2020; internal, interstate, and import operations; as well as the corresponding transport services practiced by individuals and legal entities, taxpayers or not, carried out with the equipment, supplies, and goods destined to combat, prevent, and cope with the contingency of COVID-19, an infectious disease caused by the new coronavirus (SARS-CoV-2).

Mato Grosso	LAW N° 11.177, DE 22 DE JULHO DE 2020: Implemented new regulation for the Industrial and Commercial Development Fund (FUNDEIC). LAW N° 11.157, DE 26 DE JUNHO DE 2020: Established the provision of an emergency income of R$1100 to teachers of category "V" of the State of Mato Grosso as a result of the emergency situation in the state due to the pandemic of the new coronavirus (COVID-19). – X –	LAW N° 11.177, DE 22 DE JULHO DE 2020: Implemented new regulation for the FUNDEIC.
Mato Grosso do Sul	– X –	– X –
Minas Gerais	– X –	LAW 23668, DE 26 DE JUNHO DE 2020: Allowed the Minas Gerais Research Support Foundation to stimulate scientific and technological research, development, and innovation in the health area aimed at combating the COVID-19 pandemic through public notices that provide for simplified procedures for receiving documentation, preferably through the electronic media.
Pará	LAW N° 9.032, DE 20 DE MARÇO DE 2020: Created the temporary Esperança Fund, designed to provide emergency financing to small and microentrepreneurs, as well as work cooperatives affected by the economic adversities resulting from the COVID-19 disease, caused by the new coronavirus (SARS-CoV-2), within the State of Pará. – X –	– X –
Paraíba	– X –	– X –

(Contd.)

Table 8.3 *(Contd.)*

States	Public policies for mobilizing and valuing endogenous capital	Public policies for mobilizing and valuing the externalities of business competitiveness
Paraná	– X –	LAW 20170, 7 DE ABRIL DE 2020: Authorized the Direct and Indirect Public Administration of the State of Paraná during the national emergency caused by the coronavirus, responsible for the outbreak of COVID-19, to maintain the entirety of the administrative contracts, including the frequency of payments to companies whose services have been affected with the reduction or freezing of the contracted activities, because of the public measure to combat the disease and its impacts on the public health system, as a measure that aims at the stability of the initial economic-financial balance of the contract as well as the preservation of the social labor rights.
		– X –
Pernambuco	– X –	

Piauí	– X –
Rio de Janeiro	LAW N° 8.933, DE 16 DE JULHO DE 2020: Reduced bureaucracy for the resumption of economic activity after the COVID-19 pandemic in the State of Rio de Janeiro. LAW N° 8.912, DE 29 DE JUNHO DE 2020: Authorized banks or financial institutions operating in the State of Rio de Janeiro to proceed with the contractual renegotiation or financing pause, under the criterion of advantage to the client due to the COVID-19 pandemic. LAW N° 8.910, DE 29 DE JUNHO DE 2020: Authorized the realization of a partnership between the executive branch and information technology companies to supply, in lending, microcomputers and notebooks to students from the state public network and from the Technical School Support Foundation Network while the state of public calamity persists due to the COVID-19 pandemic and make arrangements. LAW N° 8.909, DE 29 DE JUNHO DE 2020: Authorized the executive branch to institute a campaign to promote the tourism, culture, sports, leisure, and business sectors immediately after the end of the emergency situation in the public health of the State of Rio de Janeiro due to contagion and adopt measures to combat the spread arising from COVID-19 and make arrangements.	– X – LAW N° 8.933, DE 16 DE JULHO DE 2020: Reduced bureaucracy for the resumption of economic activity after the COVID-19 pandemic in the State of Rio de Janeiro. LAW N° 8.912, DE 29 DE JUNHO DE 2020: Authorized banks or financial institutions operating in the State of Rio de Janeiro to proceed with the contractual renegotiation or financing pause, under the criterion of advantage to the client due to the COVID-19 pandemic. LAW N° 8.910, DE 29 DE JUNHO DE 2020: Authorized the realization of a partnership between the executive branch and information technology companies to supply, in lending, microcomputers and notebooks to students from the state public network and from the Technical School Support Foundation Network while the state of public calamity persists due to the COVID-19 pandemic and make arrangements. LAW N° 8.887, DE 09 DE JUNHO DE 2020: Authorized the Executive Branch to use resources to implement measures to encourage the productive conversion of companies for economic and health protection to the population of Rio de Janeiro.

(Contd.)

Table 8.3 (*Contd.*)

States	Public policies for mobilizing and valuing endogenous capital	Public policies for mobilizing and valuing the externalities of business competitiveness
	LAW N° 8.905, DE 19 DE JUNHO DE 2020: Prohibited the interruption of payment and reduction of scholarships paid by the Rio de Janeiro Research Support Foundation and other scholarships paid by the State of Rio de Janeiro during the emergency situation resulting from the COVID-19 virus pandemic.	
	LAW N° 8.887, DE 09 DE JUNHO DE 2020: Authorized the Executive Branch to use resources to implement measures to encourage the productive conversion of companies for economic and health protection to the population of Rio de Janeiro.	
	LAW N° 8.886, DE 09 DE JUNHO DE 2020: Defined special procedures applicable to offshore workers affected by the COVID-19 pandemic.	
	LAW N° 8.863, DE 03 DE JUNHO DE 2020: Authorized the use of the State Funds for Culture to purchase tickets and advance tickets from cultural mechanisms.	
	LAW N° 8.824, DE 14 DE MAIO DE 2020: Authorized the Executive Branch to grant tax benefits from the tax on circulation of goods and services levied on operations and services carried out within the adoption of measures to prevent contagion to cope with the pandemic caused by COVID-19.	

Rio Grande do Norte	– X –	
Rio Grande do Sul	– X –	
Rondônia	LAW N° 4.790, DE 05 DE JUNHO DE 2020: Determined free access by telephone and mobile Internet operators to communication sites and social and streaming networks without any accounting of the customer data package and provided for the suspension of telephone and Internet services for default during the period of application of measures regarding the containment of the coronavirus (COVID-19).	LAW N° 4.790, DE 05 DE JUNHO DE 2020: Determined free access by telephone and mobile Internet operators to communication sites and social and streaming networks without any accounting of the customer data package and provided for the suspension of telephone and Internet services for default during the period of application of measures regarding the containment of the coronavirus (COVID-19)
Roraima	– X –	– X –
Santa Catarina	LAW N° 17.938, DE 4 DE MAIO DE 2020: Defined the terms of validity of authorizations and environmental licenses, within the State of Santa Catarina, as a result of the decree of public calamity due to the new coronavirus (COVID-19) pandemic.	LAW N° 17.938, DE 4 DE MAIO DE 2020: Defined the terms of validity of authorizations and environmental licenses, within the State of Santa Catarina, as a result of the decree of public calamity due to the new coronavirus (COVID-19) pandemic.

(Contd.)

Table 8.3 *(Contd.)*

States	Public policies for mobilizing and valuing endogenous capital	Public policies for mobilizing and valuing the externalities of business competitiveness
	LAW N° 17.935, DE 4 DE MAIO DE 2020: Authorized the Executive Branch to grant a partial subsidy on the interest rate on credit operations to micro- and small entrepreneurs based in the state to face the economic losses arising from the public health emergency caused by the coronavirus (COVID-19). LAW N° 17.933, DE 24 DE ABRIL DE 2020: Extended the electricity, water, sewage, and gas service payment cut-off date to December 31, 2020, within the State of Santa Catarina and established other measures in view of the health emergency caused by the pandemic of the new coronavirus (COVID-19).	LAW N° 17.935, DE 4 DE MAIO DE 2020: Authorized the Executive Branch to grant a partial subsidy on the interest rate on credit operations to micro- and small entrepreneurs based in the state to face the economic losses arising from the public health emergency caused by the coronavirus (COVID-19). LAW N° 17.933, DE 24 DE ABRIL DE 2020: Extended the electricity, water, sewage, and gas service payment cut-off date to December 31, 2020, within the State of Santa Catarina and established other measures in view of the health emergency caused by the pandemic of the new coronavirus (COVID-19).
São Paulo	– X –	– X –
Sergipe	– X –	– X –
Tocantins	– X –	– X –

Source: (Leis Estaduais, 2020).
*Federal District

Otherwise, most of the Federated States carried out actions aimed at the valorization of endogenous capital and the externalities of business competitiveness. In this regard, the States of Rio de Janeiro and Santa Catarina stand out, with the strongest intervention, with the creation of specific laws within the pandemic situation.

The State of Rio de Janeiro created nine laws for the valorization of endogenous capital, which can also be classified as valuing the externalities of business competitiveness. Among them, efforts to reduce the bureaucracy of economic activity in the post-pandemic situation can be highlighted, for example, incentives and promotion of the tourism, sport, and culture sectors. It also guaranteed incentive to the productive conversion of companies within the state territory as a form of economic protection, as well as the guarantee of payment and maintenance of the financing of scientific research.

The State of Santa Catarina, on the other hand, eased the terms for environmental licensing, granted interest rate subsidies for credit operations for micro- and small entrepreneurs within its territory, and prohibited the cutting of energy, water, and sewage services on nonpayment during the pandemic.

The remaining states adopted policies that also guaranteed minimum income to the disadvantaged population, seeking to maintain the level of consumption and demand within their states (Amapá, Bahia, and Mato Grosso), in addition to credit and other aid to micro- and small companies (Amazonas, Distrito Federal, Espírito Santo, Mato Grosso, and Paraná).

Furthermore, some states collaborated with help to public transport entrepreneurs (Distrito Federal) and guaranteed the continuity of telecommunications services even in the event of nonpayment (Rondônia). Also noteworthy is the State of Minas Gerais, which invested in scientific and technological research to develop innovations to combat COVID-19.

Evidently, many other actions were initiated by the Brazilian public administration, both by the union and the municipalities. In this paper, the actions of the Brazilian Federated States were verified, aiming at guaranteeing the resumption of the economy after overcoming the pandemic, and thus guaranteeing regional development in their territories.

8.3 Conclusions

For the economic sciences, public policies are directly related to market failures, as the means through which the public administration carries out interventions to achieve social optimums, which cannot be maximized by private agents. In this regard, the COVID-19 pandemic emerges as a challenging market failure that requires public administration to directly combat the disease, as well as to ensure that the effects of the pandemic on the economy are minimized.

Thus, it requires from the state power actions to maintain minimum levels of economic development and means to ensure economic recovery after the end of the pandemic. On this subject, at least half of the Brazilian Federated States have implemented specific public policies for mobilizing and valuing endogenous capital and the externalities of business competitiveness through the enactment of laws.

Among these states, Rio de Janeiro and Santa Catarina stand out, followed by the Distrito Federal, Amapá, Bahia, Mato Grosso, Amazonas, Espírito Santo, Paraná, Rondônia, and Minas Gerais. However, states like São Paulo and Rio Grande do Sul did not present specific laws for these types of policies, focusing exclusively on actions to combat COVID-19.

Furthermore, the controlled social distancing model carried out by the State of Rio Grande do Sul stands out, which was considered an efficient innovation in combating the pandemic. The state has one of the lowest death rates per hundred thousand inhabitants.

This study demonstrates the efforts of these subnational entities, even in the face of a federative model with many limitations like the Brazilian one, which places states with too many functions and limited resources to finance them despite the history of fiscal crises. Likewise, this study leaves open the possibility of research on the type of public policies applied by Brazilian municipalities or even the states, using other normative instruments, such as decrees.

References

1. Abrucio, F. L. and Franzese, C. (2007). Federalismo e Políticas Públicas: O Impacto das Relações Intergovernamentais no Brasil. In: *Maria de Fátima Araújo*; Ligia Beira. (Org.). Tópicos de Economia Paulista para Gestores Públicos. São Paulo: Fundap.

2. Best, N. (2011). Cooperação e Multi-level Governance: o caso do Grande Recife Consórcio de Transporte Metropolitano. 2011. 215 f. Dissertação (mestrado em administração pública e governo) - Escola de Administração de Empresas de São Paulo da Fundação Getúlio Vargas, São Paulo.

3. Constituição Federal (1988). Retrieved from: http://www.planalto. gov.br/ccivil_03/constituicao/constituicao.htm (accessed on July 20, 2020).

4. Boneti, L. W. (2007). *Políticas públicas por dentro*. Ijuí (RS): Unijuí.

5. Carvalho, M. de L., Barbosa, T. R. Da C. G. and Soares, J. B. (2010). Implementação de Política Pública: Uma abordagem Teórica e Crítica. In: *X Coloquio Internacional de Gestión Universitaria en America do Sul*. Mar del Plata.

6. Castro, J. A. de and Oliveira, M. G. de. (2014). Políticas públicas e desenvolvimento. In: Madeira, L. M. (Org.). *Avaliação de Políticas Públicas*. Porto Alegre: UFRGS/CEGOV.

7. costa, José da Silva and Nijkamp, Peter (Org.) (2009). *Compêndio de Economia Regional: Teoria, Temáticas e Políticas*. vol. 1. Coimbra: Principia.

8. Dye, T. D. (1984). *Understanding Public Policy*. Englewood Cliffs: Prentice-Hall.

9. Eastone, D. (1965). *A Framework for Political Analysis*. Englewood Cliffs: Prentice Hall.

10. Evans, P. (1989). Predatory, developmental, and other apparatuses: a comparative political economy perspective on the third world state, *Sociological Forum*, **4**(4).

11. Figueiredo, A. M. (2009). As políticas e o planeamento do desenvolvimento regional. IN: Costa, J. S., Nijkamp, P. (Org.). *Compêndio de Economia Regional: Teoria, Temáticas e Políticas*. vol. 1. Coimbra: Principia.

12. Grostein, M. D. (2001). Metrópole e expansão urbana: a persistências de processos insustentáveis, *São Paulo em Perspectiva*, **15**(1), pp. 13–19.

13. Hooghe, L. and Marks, G. (2003). Unravelling the Central State, but how? Types of Multilevel Governance, *American Political Science Review*, **97**(2), pp. 233–243.

14. Info Escola (2020). Mapas. Retrieved from: https://www.infoescola.com/geografia/mapa-do-brasil/ (accessed on July 10, 2020).

15. International Monetary Fund – FMI (2020). World Economic Outlook Update. Retrieved from: https://www.imf.org/en/Publications/WEO/Issues/2020/06/24/WEOUpdateJune2020 (accessed on July 01, 2020).

16. Instituto Brasileiro de Geografia E Estatística (IBGE) - Governo Federal do Brasil (2020). Informações Estatísticas. Retrieved from: https://www.ibge.gov.br/ (accessed on August 08, 2020).

17. Laswell, H. D. (1936). *Politics: Who Gets What, When, How*. Cleveland: Meridian Books.

18. Leis Estaduais (2020). Leis Estaduais Coronavírus. Retrieved from: https://leisestaduais.com.br/ (accessed on August 15, 2020).

19. Lima, M. J. de L. and Souza, O. T. de (2012). Tipologia de políticas públicas como instrumento de gestão, execução, coordenação e avaliação do desenvolvimento regional: uma Aplicação para o Rio Grande do Sul. Retrieved from: https://bell.unochapeco.edu.br/ revistas/index.php/grifos/article/view/2395/1449 (accessed on July 01, 2020).

20. Lima, M. J. G. de L. (2018). Proximidade e governança metropolitana: cooperação e conflitos nas políticas públicas ambientais da região metropolitana de porto alegre (RMPA). 250 f. Tese (Doutorado em Economia do Desenvolvimento) – Escola de Negócios, Pontifícia Universidade Católica do Rio Grande do Sul, Porto Alegre/RS, Brasil.

21. Lindblom, C. E. (1959). The science of muddling through, *Public Administration Review, Yale*, **19**(19), pp. 78–88.

22. Lynn, L. E. and Gould, S. G. (1980). *Designing Public Policy: A Casebook on the Role of Policy Analysis*. Santa Monica: Goodyear.

23. Mead, L. M. (1995). Public Policy: Vision, Potential, Limits, *Policy Currents, Washington*, **16**(5), pp. 1–4.

24. Painel Coronavírus (2020). Coronavírus Brasil. Retrieved from: https://covid.saude.gov.br/ (accessed on August 17, 2020).

25. Patri Políticas Públicas (2020). Cenários e perspectivas para estados. Retrieved from: https://patri.com.br/artigo/novo-coronavirus-estados (accessed on May 22, 2020).

26. Peters, G. B. (1986). *American Public Policy: Promise and Performance*, 2nd ed. Chatham: Chatham House.

27. Rolnik, R. and Klink, J. (2011). Crescimento econômico e desenvolvimento urbano: Por que nossas cidades continuam tão precárias?, *Novos Estudos*, **89**, pp. 89–109.

28. Sabatier, P. A. (1995). Political science and public policy. In: Theodoulou, S. Z. and Cahn, M. A. (Org.). *Public Policy: The Essential Readings*. New Jersey: Prentice Hall, Chap. 2, pp. 10–15.

29. Scarth, W. M. (1998). *Macroeconomics: An Introduction to Advanced Methods*. Ann Arbor: Harcourt Brace Jovanovich.

30. Secchi, L. (2013). *Políticas Públicas: Conceitos, esquemas de análise, casos práticos*, 2nd ed. São Paulo: Cengage Learning.

31. Simon, H. A. (1957). *Comportamento Administrativo*. Rio de Janeiro: USAID.

32. Soares, M. M. and Machado, J. A. (2018). *Federalismo e Políticas Pública*. Brasília: Enap.

33. Souza, C. (2006). Políticas públicas: Uma revisão da literatura, *Sociologias, Porto Alegre*, **8**(16), pp. 20–44.

34. Teixeira, E. C. (2002). O Papel das Políticas Públicas no Desenvolvimento Local e na Transformação da Realidade. Retrieved from: http://www.dhnet.org.br/dados/cursos/aatr2/a_pdf/03_aatr_pp_papel.pdf (accessed on May 28, 2017).

35. União Européia (2011). Cidades de Amanhã: desafios, visões e perspectivas. Comissão Europeia, Direção Geral da Política Regional. Bruxelas.

Chapter 9

Economic Effects of COVID-19 on Brazil in the Twenty-First Century

Iara Regina Chaves[a] and Mário Jaime Gomes de Lima[b]

[a] Porto Alegre – RGS – Brasil Dra. Qualidade Ambiental
[b] Porto Alegre – RGS – RGS – Brasil Dr. Economia
iara.chavesout@gmail.com, mariojgl@gmail.com

9.1 Introduction

Social distancing was the main public health action taken by the governors and mayors of Brazil in an effort to fight the COVID-19 pandemic. Throughout the world, social distancing has been the main course of action against the pandemic. During the Spanish influenza, it was no different, because, as verified, the cities and regions that organized social distancing measures had the best results (Correia & Verner, 2020).

Now, 100 years later, COVID-19 appears to be a disease as devastating to health as it is to the economy. The impacts of COVID-19 on the economy in the middle and long term are not yet clear (Keynes, 1964). The economic uncertainties reduce what can be foreseen and thus the investments, decreasing the expectation

Living with COVID-19: Economics, Ethics, and Environmental Issues
Edited by Chaudhery Mustansar Hussain and Gustavo Marques da Costa
Copyright © 2022 Jenny Stanford Publishing Pte. Ltd.
ISBN 978-981-4877-78-7 (Hardcover), 978-1-003-16828-7 (eBook)
www.jennystanford.com

of an economic growth (Keynes, 1964). In that sense, in order to reduce the economic uncertainties, governments have been realizing interventions to reduce the negative effects of COVID-19 on the economy, seeking to not only save lives but also save the economy, by preventing the failure of businesses, guaranteeing the maintenance of jobs and income, regardless of the future consequences of this intervention, such as the rise of public debt, for example (Bresser-Pereira, 2017). On the basis of these observations, this chapter aims to analyze the actions taken by the Brazilian government against the pandemic to reduce the economic impacts. This analysis will allow the reader to better understand the effects of the state intervention on the economy in the short term.

9.2 Overview of Influenza around the World

Flu in the twenty-first century, so far, hadn't wrought any major problems on public health, a solution having already been found by the end of the twentieth century. Vaccine for influenza H1N1 has been fulfilling its duty to immunize the population, and in cases where the vaccine had not been applied, the medication acted efficiently. Unfortunately, history tells us that influenza has been among us for a long time, as we will see now.

In 412 BC, Hippocrates related the syndrome known today as the one caused by the influenza virus. There are records of similar epidemics during the Middle Ages being present on the America continent since the fifteenth century (Souza, 2008).

To Porter (2004, p. 27), the flu was brought to the Americas by the Europeans, carried by contaminated swine on the ships. On the other hand, Aguilar (2002, p. 40) says that the flu already existed on the American continent before the arrival of the Europeans. The narrative of Aztecan chroniclers mentions the "pestilent catarrh" that spread between AD 1450 and 1456, killing a great number of people in the central part of the territory now known as Mexico.

Meanwhile, Beveridge suggests that prior to the eighteenth century, there was not adequate monitoring to allow registers to be treated as a reliable record of flu epidemics. In Brazil, the records became more precise starting from the nineteenth century.

The flu originated in the spring of 1918 in the northern hemisphere. Its origin is debatable, but the first records of the disease show it to have originated in the United States (Crosby, 1989). In March of 1918, over eight thousand workers of the Ford Motor Company, in Detroit, and many soldiers from the military base of Camp Funston/Fort Riley, in Kansas, were hospitalized after showing symptoms similar to those of the flu. In most of the cases, the disease was weak, and the patient was cured three to four days after showing the first symptoms. This encouraged the American soldiers to embark on a journey toward Europe, unknowingly carrying along a virus of the grave disease. As soon as the expeditionary American forces arrived on the French coast, the disease spread, affecting both Germans and Allies alike (Tognotti, 2003).

The emergency situation that configured itself almost simultaneously in many locations worldwide disoriented the international medic community, and medical science started to suspect that this could be a new disease. The different denominations given to that disease in the many countries where it spread were a hint of that perception: among the North Americans, it became known as the "three-day fever" or the "purple death." The term "purple" came from one of the disease symptoms, where two hours after a patient checked into the hospital, reddish-brown stains would appear on the patient's face, and a few hours later, cyanosis would start, spreading from the ears to every part of the face, to the point where it became hard to say whether the afflicted was black or white. The French called it "purulent bronchitis"; the Italians referred to it as "sand fly fever," and the Germans called it "Flanders fever" or "*blitzkatarrh*" (Crosby, 1989).

In Spain, it became known as "*la dançarina*" (the dancer), in Portugal, as "*a pneumónica*" (the pneumatic), and in other countries as the Spanish flu or influenza (Diário de Notícias, 23 set. 1918, p. 1). The name "Spanish" came from the fact that on Spanish lands, there were no secrets kept about the damages caused by the disease, as opposed to many countries that sought to smooth over the impact of the pandemic on their societies (D'ávila, 1993; Kolata, 2002).

The name "Spanish" had political roots, given the neutral position Spain had during World War I and a demonstration of sympathy by a faction of the Spanish government toward the Germans, leading to an English initiative to attribute the disease to Spain to gain political amplitude (D'ávila, 1993).

The Spanish flu occurred in the twentieth century and saw three waves between March 1918 and May 1919. The first (March–August 1918), although extremely contagious, was deemed weak, for it caused relatively few deaths. Till then, there were confirmed cases only in the United States and Europe. Starting from the second wave (August 1918–February 1919), there was severe aggravation. During that period, the disease spread to India, South Asia, Japan, China, Africa, and Middle and South America. In all these countries, it caused an enormous number of deaths. The third wave (February–May of 1919), although more lethal than the first, led to fewer deaths than the second (Souza, 2008).

From May 1919, an epidemic disease whose diagnosis was uncertain assailed Europe and Africa. Only by the end of July did London confirm that it was in fact the influenza (its fourth wave) and that it had spread to many places of Europe. It probably traveled the rest of the world in the next eight months. Ultimately, it ended up killing between 50 and 100 million people worldwide, becoming the biggest medicine enigma of the time (Goulart, 2005).

9.3 The History of Influenza in Brazil

In Brazil, the epidemic arrived in September 1918. The English boat *Demerara*, coming from Lisbon, Spain, disembarked the sick at Recife, Salvador e Rio de Janeiro (capital of Brazil at the time). In the same month, sailors that served in the army in Dakar, on the Atlantic coast of Africa, disembarked the sick in the port of Recife. A little more than two weeks later, there were cases of the flu in other cities, like Nordeste and São Paulo (Fiocruz, 2020).

The Brazilian authorities did not give the case the importance it needed, even after the arrival of news from Portugal about the suffering caused by the flu pandemic in Europe. They believed, at the time, that the ocean would prevent the arrival of the disease to the country, a belief that was quickly proved to be wrong. People were afraid to go out. In São Paulo, especially those who had the means, left the city, fleeing to the interior, where the disease had not arrived yet. In the face of the lack of known methods to prevent the contagion or to cure the sick, authorities only recommended that agglomerations should be avoided (Fiocruz, 2020).

It is estimated that between October and December 1918, the period officially established as that of the pandemic, 65% of the population fell sick. In Rio de Janeiro itself, 14,348 deaths were registered. In São Paulo, another 2000 people had died. Between 1918 and 1920, approximately 35,000 people had died across the country, including the then elected president Rodrigues Alves (Fiocruz, 2nd ed, 2020).

9.4 The Influenza and the Brussels International Finance Conference

According to Smith (2020), this conference was proposed by the then just formed United Nations. It happened in September 1920 and had representatives from both the banking and business sectors from over 40 countries. The results of the conference were analyzed in 1922, with reports of over 20 countries about the economic measures taken, and published as a long and detailed report. However, they do not possess any reference to the Spanish flu— neither about its economic impact nor about any measures the governments had taken about it. The US report referred to it, but not directly, when it said "[I]n the beginning of 1919, after a short period of falling prices and commercial contraction. ..." Shortly after, the report also refers to "a period of expansion, inflation and speculation, the kind of never seen before. ...."

The virus that had just killed millions of people throughout the world was not considered to have any economic relevance to the present or the future by the politicians of the time!

9.5 The Return of the Virus in the Twenty-First Century

On March 11 of this year (2020), the World Health Organization (WHO) decreed that the world was facing a pandemic—of the new coronavirus (COVID-19). In a report disclosed in September 2019, and as such, before the first cases of the disease being officially reported, the WHO alerted that:

> . . . The world is not prepared for a fast-moving, virulent respiratory pathogen pandemic. The 1918 global influenza pandemic sickened one third of the world population and killed as many as 50 million people - 2.8% of the total population. If a similar contagion occurred today with a population four times larger and travel times anywhere in the world less than 36 hours, 50 - 80 million people could perish. In addition to tragic levels of mortality, such a pandemic could cause panic, destabilize national security and seriously affect the global economy and trade.[1]

On December 31, 2019, the WHO was notified about the occurrence of a pneumonic outbreak in the city of Wuhan, Hubei Province, China. The etiological agent was quickly identified as a new coronavirus: SARS-CoV-2. The outbreak began in a seafood and living animal market and as of the time this book is going to the press, the animal reservoir is unknown.[2]

The first meeting of the Emergency Committee about the new coronavirus outbreak in China convened by the WHO under the International Health Regulations (2005) occurred on January 23, 2020. In this meeting, there was no agreement on whether the event was indeed a public health emergency of international concern (PHEIC).[3] During the second meeting, on January 30, the growing

---

[1] As mentioned in the Global Preparedness Monitoring Board Report 2019. Available at: <https://apps.who.int/gpmb/annual_report.htm>.

[2] Zhu, N., Zhang, D., Wang, W., Li, X., Yang, B., Song, J., et al. (2019). A novel coronavirus from patients with pneumonia in China, N. Engl. J. Med., [Internet] [cited 2020 Mar 4], **382**, pp. 727–733. Available at: <http://doi.org/10.1056/NEJMoa2001017>.

[3] World Health Organization (2020). Statement on the second meeting of the International Health Regulations (2005) Emergency Committee regarding the outbreak of novel coronavirus (2019-nCoV), [Internet]. Geneva: World Health

number of cases and countries that reported confirmed cases led to the declaration of the outbreak as a PHEIC.[4]

On February 2020, in accordance with WHO best practices in naming new infectious human diseases, the sickness caused by the new coronavirus was given the name COVID-19, referring to the virus type and the year the pandemic began: coronavirus disease 2019.[5]

The approach to the disease won't be a matter of just the actual capability of governments to deliver results but also of the perception of citizens about government action, being, in that way, about the realm of action that transcends technical aspects and demands political competence (Christensen et al., 2016).

The first case of COVID-19 in Brazil was confirmed on February 26, 2020. On March 3, there were 488 suspected cases reported, 2 were confirmed, and 240 reports were discarded, with no evidence of local transmission. The first two confirmed cases were males, residing in the city of São Paulo, who had returned from a trip to Italy (Croda & Garcia, 2020).

The scant scientific knowledge in the world about the new coronavirus, its high speed of dissemination, and its capacity to cause deaths in vulnerable populations create uncertainties about what should be done and what is the best strategy to be used across the world to face the pandemic. In Brazil, this is even more challenging in the context of great social inequality, with vulnerable populations living in precarious housing and sanitation conditions,

---

Organization, [cited 2020 Mar 4]. Available at: https://www.who.int/news-room/detail/30-01-2020-statement-on-the-second-meeting-of-the-international-health-regulations-(2005)-emergency-committee-regarding-the-outbreak-of-novel-coronavirus-(2019-ncov).

[4]World Health Organization (2020). Statement on the second meeting of the International Health Regulations (2005) Emergency Committee regarding the outbreak of novel coronavirus (2019-nCoV), [Internet]. Geneva: World Health Organization, [cited 2020 Mar 4]. Available at: https://www.who.int/news-room/detail/30-01-2020-statement-on-the-second-meeting-of-the-international-health-regulations-(2005)-emergency-committee-regarding-the-outbreak-of-novel-coronavirus-(2019-ncov).

[5]World Health Organization (2020). Novel coronavirus (2019-nCoV): situation report – 22, [Internet]. Geneva: World Health Organization, [cited 2020 Mar 4]. Available at: https://www.who.int/docs/default-source/coronaviruse/situation-reports/20200211-sitrep-22-ncov.pdf?sfvrsn=fb6d49b1_2.

without access to water and in a situation of agglomeration (Werneck & Carvalho, 2020).

The success of the measures adopted to confront the disease, however, is contingent upon effective governmental coordination (IPEA, 2020).

9.6 Economic Crisis in the EU in Times of the Pandemic

The new coronavirus pandemic has profoundly affected the economic trajectory of all countries in the world. The most recent forecast of the International Monetary Fund (IMF) is that the world gross domestic product (GDP) will fall by 4.9% this year. Brazil, as well as the rest of the world, will suffer this impact, already observed with the survey of the GDP for the first quarter, which fell by 1.5% in relation to the previous quarter, and it is estimated that the fall in the second quarter, characterized by the deepening of social distance measures in response to the pandemic, will approach 10%. Under the assumption that the process of gradually easing restrictions on mobility and the functioning of economic activities that began in June will continue, the gradual recovery of GDP is projected in the third and fourth quarters. The projected drop for the year is 6%, but the recovery path in the second half will leave a carry-over of almost 2% for 2021, whose projected growth is 3.6% (IPEA, 2020).

In accordance with the Institute for Applied Economic Research (IPEA, 2020), as has been common in forecasts released recently, the IMF warns of the high degree of uncertainty surrounding its projections. Positive risks arise, among other factors, from the possibility of a vaccine being developed in a shorter time than the one estimated on the basis of past pandemics. Furthermore, additional economic policy measures may accelerate the recovery of economic activity. On the negative side, the increase in mobility and resultant neglect of social distance measures involves an overwhelming risk of new contagion waves and the need to reverse the process, depressing activity again and putting financial conditions back in the restrictive field.

The IMF also highlights the geopolitical tensions and risks associated with international trade, which should drop by 12% in the year, with an 8% growth projected in 2021.

The fall and recovery of the American stock market since the arrival of the pandemic was accompanied by a sharp rise and a subsequent decline in volatility: the VIX index reached 80 points on March 16, almost 20 points more than that observed at the height of the financial crisis in 2008. After that, it fell, averaging 30 points in May and June—still 50% higher than the 2019 average.

The global monetary stimulus has been astonishing: interest rates are practically zero in the United States and negative in Europe and Japan. Policies for quantitative expansion have been intensely used. In the monetary expansion after the international crisis of 2008, the Federal Reserve System (Fed) increased its balance sheet by about USD 2 trillion in the course of almost three years, through the acquisition of public and mortgage-backed securities (Fig. 9.1). In the current pandemic phase, there was an even greater increase, on the order of USD 3 trillion in just three months, between March and June of this year, with the assets acquired by the Fed now also

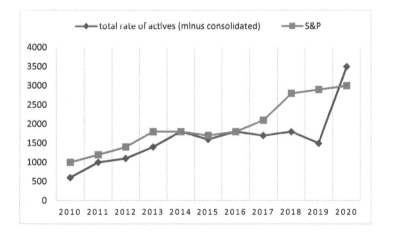

Figure 9.1 US Federal assets (in trillion USDs) and S&P 500 Index (in points). *Source*: Federal Reserve Bank of St. Louis. Elaboration: DIMAC/IPEA. S&P 500 Index of shares traded on the New York Stock Exchange (apud IPEA, 2020).

including private corporate bonds. A similar move was followed by central banks in the Euro Area and Japan (IPEA, 2020).

In line with IPEA (2020), in China, industrial production increased again in the year-on-year comparison (4.2% per year, on average, in April and May), after strong falls, of 13.5% on average, in January and February 2020. Retail sales, on the other hand, still show negative (but decreasing) rates in the interannual comparison, indicating the possible presence of restrictions on mobility and the impact of consumers' loss of income, combined with greater caution in view of the uncertainties that remain.

In the United States, industrial production grew by 1.4% in May 2020 (after falling 16.5% in March–April 2020), while retail sales increased by 16.8%, reflecting the support of household income through the government's money transfer programs. June's prior disclosures from the purchasing manager indexes point to the continuation of the recovery movement, with the American industry indicator at 49.6 points and the Euro Area indicator at 46.9 points, growths of 37% and 40%, respectively, in relation to the slope, in April. In the services sector, the recovery is more striking, but starting from much lower levels than in the industry. In China, more advanced in normalizing the functioning of the economy, the (preliminary) indicators for both industry and services are already above 50 points, indicating the expansion of economic activity.

The external environment is challenging. The ample international liquidity and the return of the risk voracity contribute to better financial conditions. The downturn in the world economy will be profound, but for a short period, if the IMF's forecasts are confirmed. The stimulation of economic policies on a global scale is significant, specifically for the Brazilian economy. In addition to the expected resumption of foreign capital flows, the recovery in activity levels in developed countries and China should keep the foreign market in a position to absorb Brazilian exports: the prices of commodities relevant to Brazil, such as agricultural products and minerals, had a lower drop than the average of commodities, which is greatly influenced by the price of oil, which fell by almost 50% in relation to the last quarter of 2019. The price of soybeans fell by 8%, compared to a reduction average of 4.3% for agricultural products;

Table 9.1 Projections for GNP growth and unemployment rate

	GNP		Unemployment rate	
	2020	**2021**	**2020**	**2021**
India	1.9%	7.4%	—	—
South Korea	−1.2%	3.4%	4.5%	4.5%
Australia	−6.7%	6.1%	7.6%	8.9%
New Zealand	−7.2%	5.9%	9.2%	6.8%
Spain	−8%	4.3%	20.8%	17.5%
Portugal	−8%	5%	13.9%	8.7%

Source: SEBRAE, 2020.

iron ore had an increase of 4.4% in the same comparison, while for the set of metallic commodities the fall was 11% (IPEA, 2020).

According to the IMF, all the countries selected here will see a drop in gross national product (GNP) this year, except India, which is expected to expand by 1.9%. The biggest retractions should occur in Spain and Portugal (−8%). In 2021, India is expected to lead the rise in GNP (+7.4%). In relation to the unemployment rate, Spain is expected to register the highest rate in 2020 (20.8%), followed by Portugal (13.9%), as shown in Fig. 9.2, under the impact of COVID-19 (SEBRAE, 2020)

9.7 Economic crisis in Brazil in Times of the Pandemic

According to the IPEA (2020), in Brazil, the expectation of a gradual resumption of demand, combined with the idle capacity present in most productive sectors and the reduction in labor and rental costs, allows one to project a trajectory without major changes in the prices of services and free goods. The DIMAC/IPEA group forecasts the inflation (measured by the IPCA)[6] at the year end at 1.8%.

---

[6] IPCA – Índice Nacional de Preços ao Consumidor Amplo – IPCA que tem por objetivo medir a inflação de um conjunto de produtos e serviços comercializados no varejo, referentes ao consumo pessoal das famílias. Available at: https://www.ibge.gov.br/estatisticas/economicas/precos-e-custos/9256-indice-nacional-de-precos-ao-consumidor-amplo.html?=&t=o-que-e.

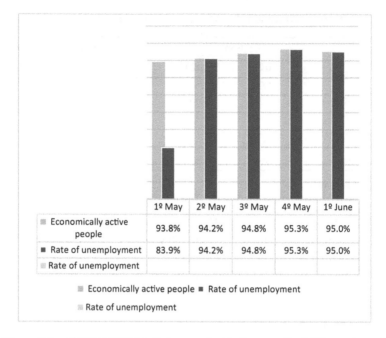

	1º May	2º May	3º May	4º May	1º June
▩ Economically active people	93.8%	94.2%	94.8%	95.3%	95.0%
■ Rate of unemployment	83.9%	94.2%	94.8%	95.3%	95.0%
▩ Rate of unemployment					

▩ Economically active people ■ Rate of unemployment

▩ Rate of unemployment

Figure 9.2 PNAD COVID-19: Labor market indicators (in 1000 people and in %). *Source*: PNAD COVID-19/IBGE.

Brazil also felt the effects of the crisis as strongly as the rest of the world. The first-quarter GDP fell by 1.5%, already reflecting the impact of COVID-19 and the first social distance measures adopted since the second half of March. April seemed to show bottoming out, with strong declines in relation to March in industry (−18.8%), commerce (−17.5%), and services (−11.7%) according to monthly surveys of the Brazilian Institute of Geography and Statistics (IBGE, 2020).

The occupation in April 2020 reflected the contraction of economic activity, with a drop of 3.4% in relation to the same period of 2019—after a monthly average of the annual rate of growth of 2% in the previous 12 months. In comparison, the real mass of income from work fell by 0.8%, compared to a monthly average of the 2.2% interannual variation in the previous 12 months. The unemployment rate in the moving quarter up to April was 12.6%, 0.4% more than in March (not seasonally adjusted) and 0.1% more than a year earlier, registering the first positive change after 20 months of decline as of the last quarter of 2017. The "monthly payment" of the National Continuous Household Survey (PNAD Continuous)[7] reveals that, specifically for April, the unemployment rate would have increased to 13.1%, compared to 12.8% in February. This rate could have been even higher had it not been for the drop in the participation rate, from 61.9% in February to 59% in April 2019—in this case, the lowest participation rate since the beginning of the survey (IPEA, 2020).

According to the IPEA (2020), the drop in the participation rate represents the restrictions resulting from the strong reduction in economic activity and the physical limitation itself in the search for work.

9.7.1 COVID-19 and the Labor Market

According to PNAD COVID-19 (IBGE, 2020), in the fourth week of May, out of the 74.6 million people of working age who were out of the labor force, 25.7 million (or 34.4% of the total) did not look for a job but stated that they would like to work (the discouraged ones). It is worth mentioning that the pandemic was probably the main factor that led people who would like to work not to look for a job in the reference week; according to IBGE, of this contingent of people, 17.7 million stated that they had not sought employment due to the pandemic or due to lack of work in the locality.

The indicator of adherence to social distance, as shown, peaked at the end of March and dropped systematically from that point on, reflecting the ever-reducing adherence to the rules of isolation. The degree of rigidity of the legal measures of social distancing, according to the indicator developed by the IPEA, reduced only slightly in April and increased again in May. On June 20, the in-loco social isolation index was just under 40% while the index of legal distance measures was approximately 55%.

---

[7] National Household Sample Survey Continues (Continuous PNAD) aims to monitor the quarterly fluctuations and the evolution, in the short, medium, and long terms, of the workforce and other necessary information for the study of the socioeconomic development of the country.

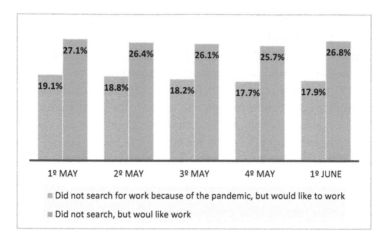

Figure 9.3 PNAD COVID-19: Effect of the pandemic on the demand for work (in 1000 people and in %). *Source*: PNAD COVID-19/IBGE.

The decline in the social isolation index seems consistent with the observation derived from PNAD COVID-19, that the increase in unemployment in recent weeks has reflected much more the increase in the labor force (i.e., in the number of people looking for employment) than the drop in occupation. Corroborating this perception, while the level of employment decreased by 0.3% between the first week of May and the first week of June, the number of people in the workforce expanded by 1.3% (IPEA, 2020).

We present in Fig. 9.2 the percentage of employed persons and economically active (EA) persons and unemployment rates per week from data collected in the months of May and June 2020.

In Fig. 9.3, we will show the number of people who did not seek employment but would like to work (the discouraged) and the number who did not seek employment because of the pandemic but would like to work and finally the percentage of unemployed people.

According to IBGE (2020), the workforce and its performance between 12 July and 18 July 2020 is according to Chart 9.1.

Regarding the income of employed persons (Chart 9.1), 36% had a lower income than that normally received. This drop in income is due to the public policies that allowed entrepreneurs to reduce the workload and suspend the employment contract through

Chart 9.1 Income of employed persons during COVID-19

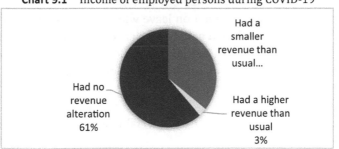

Source: IBGE, 2020.[8]

Provisional Measure (MP) 936/2020 (Emergency Employment and Income Maintenance Program)[9] effective from April 1, 2020, authorizing employers to reduce employees' wages and working hours during the coronavirus pandemic to preserve jobs. In both cases, the government will compensate part of the loss in the workers' remuneration through the social security benefit, which is an amount that the Federal Government will pay to the employee in the case of proportional reduction of the working day and salary and temporary suspension of the employment contract. The benefit amount was based on the monthly unemployment insurance amount to which the employee would be entitled. The amount will depend on what change was made in the employment contract. The amount paid by the Federal Government will not exceed the ceiling of unemployment insurance, which is R$1813[10] (i.e., USD 349.33).

Other factors that have prevented a more significant increase in the unemployment rate have been the possibilities of remote work in several productive activities and the use of temporary leave from work, with maintenance of the occupation. According to the survey, in the last week of May, there were 8.8 million people working

---

[8]https://covid19.ibge.gov.br/pnad-covid/trabalho.php

[9]MP 936/2020 aims to preserve employment and income, guarantee the continuity of work and business activities, and reduce the social impact resulting from the consequences of the state of public calamity and public health emergency. Provisional Measure 936/20 creates unemployment insurance benefits in a supplementary format of up to 70% of wages to compensate workers' wage reductions.

[10]USD 5.19 (on April 1, 2020).

remotely in the country (home office or telework). The percentage of persons employed and not on leave who worked remotely in the total employed population and not on leave varied between 13.1% and 13.4% in May. With regard to employed persons who were temporarily removed from work, there were 17.6 million workers in this condition in the last week of May, 14.6 million of whom (or 82.8% of the total) were in this condition due to social distance (in quarantine or isolation, under social distance, or on collective vacations).

A small portion of the population worked remotely, which meant 8.2 million people. The level of education of people in remote work was fundamentally marked by those workers with a higher level of education, where people with higher education or postgraduate education represented 31.9%, followed by those with incomplete higher education or complete high school (5.9%), those with complete elementary school or incomplete high school (1.2%), and persons without instruction or incomplete elementary school (0.3%). These figures reflect the situation in June 2020 (IBGE, 2020).

The number of households that received emergency aid (AE) from the Brazilian government was 43%. The average income from emergency assistance received by households was of R$881 (USD 169.75), with the majority being of the population from the north and northeast of the country.

The breakdown of data by region show that for the northeast and the north, the effect of AE was even more significant, not only because the value of this emergency benefit was greater in these regions, but also because in these locations the average of yields is lower (Table 9.2). In the north, the average AE (R$936.16) was 17% higher than the average received by self-employed workers (R$801.46). Regarding domestic work (R$616.73), the assistance was 52% higher. In the northeast, comparisons show that the average aid received (R$907.37) was 46% higher than the income of self-employed workers (R$616.6) and 87% higher than the income of domestic workers (R$485.76).

In the analysis of households per decile of income per capita (Table 9.3), it appears that 72% of the households in the lowest income decile obtained the benefit. This proportion rises to 88.7%

Table 9.2 SE and income from work as on May 2020 (in R$)

	Actual average income actually received by all employed persons with income from work			
	Average AE income received by households	**All busy**	**Domestic workers**	**Self-employed**
Brazil	846.50	1898.86	698.37	1092.12
Norte	936.16	1495.27	616.73	801.46
Nordeste	907.37	1319.33	485.76	619.6
Sudeste	790.58	2125.84	775.52	1264.49
Sul	771.89	2098.87	788.94	1469.92
Centro-Oeste	794.12	1167.55	788.91	1263.52

Source: PNAD COVID-19/IBGE.
Elaboration: Conjuncture Group of the Directorate of Studies and Macroeconomic Policies (DIMAC) of IPEA (apud IPEA, 2020).

in the following decile and gradually decreases until reaching 5% in the highest income decile.

The weight of the EA in per capita household income can be analyzed in Table 9.4. For the households of the lowest income percent, the EA meant a significant portion of the income. In the case of the lowest percent, it can be observed that the aid represented

Table 9.3 Households benefited by AE in each decile (income in R$)

Income decile*	Upper limit of per capita household income (in R$)	Total households (in thousands)	Total households benefited (in thousands)	%
1	56.62	6780	4872	72
2	233.18	5047	4074	80.7
3	348.83	5261	3570	67.9
4	499.88	4698	2902	61.8
5	645.54	7208	3506	48.6
6	832.65	6157	2575	41.0
7	1044.98	5095	1603	31.5
8	1440	10,658	1635	15.3
9	2275.13	8184	1106	13.5
10		8935	461	5.2
		68,023	23,304	38.7

Source: PNAD COVID-19/IBGE. Elaboration: DIMAC/IPEA Business Group (apud IPEA, 2020).
[†] The 1st decile is the cutoff point for 10% of the lowest data, that is, the 10th percentile.

Table 9.4 Participation of the EA in per capita household percent

Income decile	Per capita household income (in R$)	Household income per capita excluding the EA (in R$)	Difference in per capita household income due to the EA (in R$)	EA participation in the household income per capita (%)
1	238.03	10.64	227.39	95.53
2	352.85	146.08	206.77	56.8
3	453.69	295.77	157.92	34.81
4	554.72	414.47	140.25	25.28
5	672.64	553.40	119.24	17.73
6	826.83	729.71	97.12	11.75
7	1014.27	938.08	76.19	7.51
8	1231.05	1184.99	46.06	3.74
9	1823.75	1785.40	38.35	2.1
10	4661.66	4646.14	15.52	0.33
	1189.79	1078.31	111.48	9.37

Source: PNAD COVID-19/IBGE. Prepared by DIMAC/IPEA (apud IPEA, 2020).

almost the total per capita household income (about 95%). In the second- and third-lowest income percent, the EA represented more than a third of the household income per capita (59% and 35%, respectively). Inward from the other lower income percent, the participation of the EA in household income was also substantial.

9.7.2 The Different Sectors of the Economy and COVID-19

According to the IPEA (2020), the Cielo index of nominal retail revenue, which compares the weekly sales of different segments of the trade in relation to the precrisis period, shows that the strong drops in sales at the end of March and April have been giving way to less negative variations in all segments. In this recovery, the segments of other nondurable consumer goods and clothing stand out. In furniture and appliances, construction materials, and other consumer durables, the variations are already positive.

As shown in Chart 9.2, drugstore and pharmacy retailers had a very large growth (36.1%) in the week from 3/15 to 3/21 of 2020, falling again in the following weeks.

The same did not happen in the retail of super- and hypermarkets, which in the week from 3/15 to 3/21 of 2020 had an increase of 57.8% and remained high, although not at the same level, closing the week from 6/14 to 6/20 with an increase of 18.2%.

In the industry, preliminary indicators point to the beginning of a reversal of the strong fall in April 2020. There are indicators of resumption of production in sectors such as the automobile industry, clothing, machinery and equipment, and information technology and electronics. On the other hand, it is estimated that the food industry, which grew in April (+3.3% in relation to March) amid the generalized retraction of the other segments of the manufacturing industry, fell in May (−1.3%).

Another important point for analyzing the resumption in the industry is the consumption of electricity by the industrial sector, which is one of the variables that point to the resumption of production. After a sharp drop in April 2020, there was an almost general recovery in May. In June (average of the first twelve days), some sectors, the most affected in April, maintained their growth, while in others, there was a slight decrease compared to May.

Chart 9.2 Cielo retail index: Nondurable consumer goods—variation in nominal revenue in relation to February (equivalent days) of 2020, with calendar adjustment (%)

Pharmacies and drugstores		Super- and hypermarkets	
3/1–3/7	4.5%	3/1–3/7	3.3%
3/8–3/14	15%	3/8–3/14	11.3%
3/15–3/21	36.1%	3/15–3/21	57.8%
3/22–3/28	−16.2%	3/22–3/28	5.7%
3/29–4/4	−11.2%	3/29–4/4	11.8%
4/5–4/11	−8.9%	4/5–4/11	10.8%
4/12–4/18	−13.9%	4/12–4/18	20.5%
4/19–4/25	−15%	4/19–4/25	22.7%
4/26–5/2	−10%	4/26–5/2	19.9%
5/3–5/9	−2.9%	5/3–5/9	16.5%
5/10–5/16	−5.2%	5/10–5/16	8.6%
5/17–5/23	−10.2%	5/17–5/23	12.9%
5/24–5/30	−13.2%	5/24–5/30	7%
5/31–6/6	−1.5%	5/31–6/6	15.7%
6/9–6/13	−0.9%	6/9–6/13	18.1%
6/14–6/20	−7.1%	6/14–6/20	18.2%

Source: Modified from IPEA, 2020.

The industry's confidence indexes in June 2020, by the surveys by both the Brazilian Institute of Economics (IBRE) of the Getúlio Vargas Foundation and the National Confederation of Industry (CNI), showed an important recovery. In the case of the IBRE survey, it advanced to 76.6 points, compared to 61.4 points in May, reflecting an improvement both in the current situation index (77.8% in June compared to 68.6% in May) and in the index expectation, which went from 54.9% to 75.5% in the period. In the CNI, where neutrality corresponds to 50% points, the index went from 34.7% points to 41.2% points (IPEA, 2020).

Part of the confidence presented by the industry area is due to the government's income transfer program that took place through AE,[11] which began to take shape as of second half of April 2020, causing an important impact on sales. The National Treasury has already made disbursements of R$ 95.6 billion through this program, which does not mean that this amount has already reached families. Assuming that these payments refer to two months' worth of the aid, which would give R$47.8 billion per month, one can compare it with an estimate of the pre-COVID-19 income of the target population of the program. The mass income from the main job received monthly by persons employed in the informal sector (employees without a license and employers not in the National Register of Legal Entities [CNPJ] and self-employed persons not in the CNPJ) in the quarter ended in February 2020, before the crisis worsened, was R$49.7 billion. The latest forecast of the total spending on AE is R$152.6 billion, which is equivalent to about 2.2% of the projected GDP for the year (IPEA, 2020).

9.8 Small and Medium-Sized Enterprises

We will now deal with the impact on small and medium-sized companies, which are the most affected by the fragile or no short- and medium-term planning, basically in terms of the necessary working capital. These companies deserve to be highlighted in this study because they employ a number of workers who do not need to have any major specialization.

In 2019, 16% of the adult Brazilian population was part of the "established entrepreneurs." Brazil was in 2nd place in the ranking of the 50 countries participating in the survey that year. This is an indication that the relative participation of the Brazilian population in conducting small businesses (in the CNPJ or not) in the country is high (SEBRAE, 2020).

---

[11]Emergency aid is financial benefit granted by the Federal Government for informal workers, individual microentrepreneurs, and the self-employed and unemployed and aims to provide emergency protection during the period of coping with the crisis caused by the coronavirus pandemic (COVID-19) amounting to R$600, or USD 115.061 (USD 1 = R$5.19 as of 4/4/2020). From <https://www.gov.br/cidadania/pt-br/servicos/auxilio-emergencial>.

SEBRAE conducted a survey from 6/25 to 6/30 of 2020 in the universe of 17.2 million small businesses with the following sample size and distribution: 6470 respondents from all 26 states and Federal District, composed of 57% MEI, 38% ME, and 5% EPP (*size declared in the survey), with a sample error of ±1% for national results, with a confidence interval of 95%.

The survey presented data such as the drop in revenue, companies that requested financing from financial institutions, and the return of requests, both positive and negative, among other information.

We will now present the data considered relevant for the analysis of the economic recovery of companies of this size

Chart 9.3 represents the turnover of small businesses in the precrisis period of the COVID-19 from 3/23 to 6/30 of 2020 by region and in Brazil.

The chart shows that the southeast region has −53% of revenue recovery, the lowest index, lower than the average of Brazil; the southern states have the same percentage as of Brazil, of −51%; and the other regions have the recovery slightly higher, although the pace of recovery is slow, in the form of a ramp.

Chart 9.3 Revenue in relation to the precrisis period

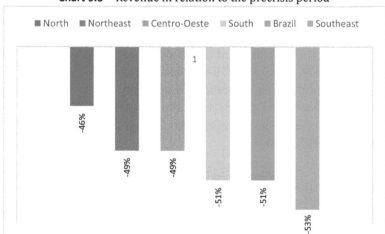

Source: SEBRAE, 2020.

The fifth edition of the survey "The Impact of the Coronavirus Pandemic on Small Businesses" shows that the lack of guarantees was one of the main reasons informed by the entrepreneurs for not being able to obtain credit from financial institutions. Therefore, the Guarantee Fund is a mechanism used to grant guarantees complementary to the contracting of credit operations to finance investments by companies with financial institutions (SEBRAE, 2020).

In times of turbulence in the economy, small companies need financial support to remain active in the market. However, this is one of the main negative impacts, as they are hardly able to guarantee the capital that is being requested from financial institutions, as shown by the research carried out by SEBRAE, demonstrating the difficulty of obtaining credit for their business.

Figure 9.4 shows that in the fifth edition of the survey, there was an increase in companies requesting a loan, going from 7.9 million in the fourth edition to 6.7 million in the fifth edition. This proportion is higher among micro- and small companies by 57%.

Regarding the return of the loan request to financial institutions, it is observed that a few companies obtained a loan. Only 1.4 million, that is, 18% of the total research population, had their request

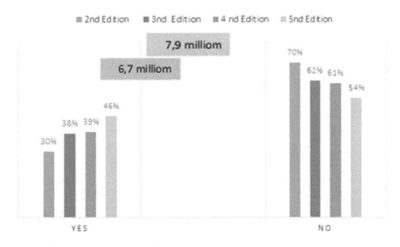

Figure 9.4 The number of companies that applied for a loan. *Source*: SEBRAE, 2020.

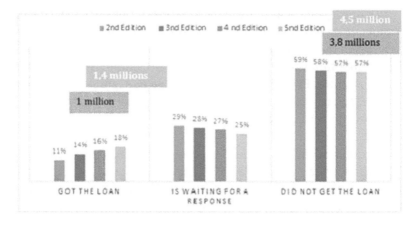

Figure 9.5 Status of loan applications to financial institutions. *Source*: SEBRAE, 2020.

fulfilled; 4.5 million (59%) failed to obtain financing; and in the 5th edition, 29% are still keeping their request back (Fig. 9.5).

Figure 9.6 shows us the reasons that entrepreneurs in this niche would seek bank loans, drawing a relationship between 2019 and 2020. Of the entrepreneurs surveyed in 2019, 50% believed that they did not need a loan, the number reducing to 28% in 2020. In 2019, 6% of the entrepreneurs believed that they would not

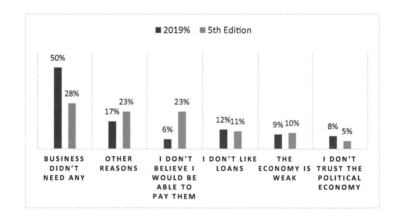

Figure 9.6 Answers to the question, why haven't you tried bank loans since the beginning of the crisis? *Source*: SEBRAE, 2020.

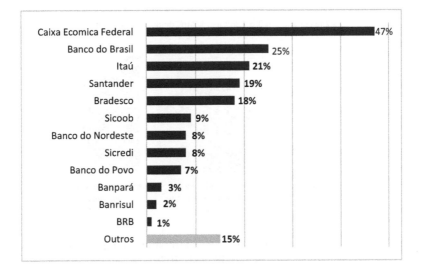

Figure 9.7   Financial institutions sought for loans. *Source*: SEBRAE, 2020.

be able to repay the requested loan, and this number increased to 23% in 2020. In 2019, 9% of those surveyed believed the economy was weak; very little changed in 2020, with this percentage increasing to 10%. And in 2019, 8% of the entrepreneurs said they did not trust the economic policy, the percentage reducing 5% in 2020.

Regarding the financial institutions that entrepreneurs sought loans from, the most sought after in the 5th edition of the survey were government banks, as shown in Fig. 9.7.

Of the financial institutions that were sought for a loan as a means of paying off debts and remaining in the market, 72% of entrepreneurs sought government institutions; the remaining 28% sought loans from private or cooperative institutions.

Figure 9.8 shows the situation of the companies in relation to the change in their functioning and whether they have ceased to function.

As can be seen, more companies that were stopped have started to work again. The "temporary interruption" drops from 43% to 29%. The number of companies that closed their activities totally increased from 3% to 4% (a barely perceptible increase).

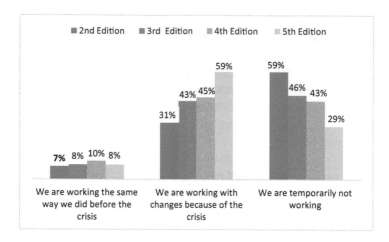

Figure 9.8 Answers to the question, did your company change its operations with the crisis? *Source*: SEBRAE, 2020.

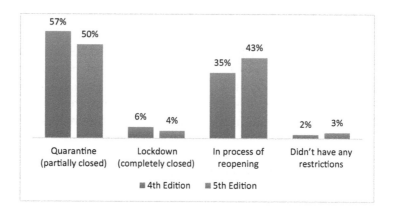
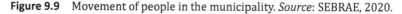

Figure 9.9 Movement of people in the municipality. *Source*: SEBRAE, 2020.

Figure 9.9 shows the information as a relation to the restriction of movement of people in the municipalities studied, from 5/29 to 6/2 and from 6/25 to 6/30 of 2020.

About 30 days after the last survey, it was noted that taking into account the national scenario, the movement of people was reduced from 57% to 50% because of quarantine and partial closure. In the same periods, the movement of the people was reduced was from 6% to 4% because of total closure (lockdown); in the process of reopening, the movement of the people increased from 35% to 43%, and the number of those who faced no restriction on movement increased from 2% to 3%.

In June 2020, the country had reached the figures of 101,149 deaths and 3,035,422 infections caused by the new coronavirus since the beginning of the pandemic. The state with the highest number of deaths was São Paulo (25,114), followed by Rio de Janeiro (14,080) and Ceará (7954). The figures from the Ministry of Health are in line with the most recent bulletin from the National Council of Health Secretaries, which created a platform to record data on the new coronavirus in the country after the Ministry of Health started to disclose, at the beginning July 2020, the figures in less detail. After the controversy caused by the change and a decision by the Federal Supreme Court on the matter, the Ministry of Health started to release the complete numbers.

9.9 Final Considerations

In view of the data presented, we observed that some lessons in relation to the Spanish flu and COVID-19 were not learned, mainly in terms of the real severity, the speed of spread, and the mortality in the population caused by the virus. Neither people not governments understand the need for social distancing to minimize the degree of contagion of the disease, guided by those who can better guide science, the medical profession, and virology students.

As of August 9, 2020, the number of deaths in the United States was 161,964; in Brazil 101,049; in Mexico 52,006; and in the world 728,612.

In relation to public policies, we observe that the world did not consider it to be a pandemic with a high degree of mortality and diverse impacts, including on the economy, until it was too late. The same was the case with the Spanish flu. At one of the main world conferences, the Brussels Conference held in September 1920, where representatives of the business and banking sectors from more than 40 countries were present, the Spanish flu and its consequences found literally no mention.

Brazil sought palliative measures to try to reverse the economic scenario of falling sales and production, but with little representation, as shown by the GDP forecast figures and the resumption of industries.

Despite the high demand for loans by small companies from banks managed by the government, these were not approved according to the SEBRAE survey, which indicated that 4.5 million entities did not have their credit approved, which possibly resulted in numerous companies closing their doors for ever, and it is unlikely that the economy will be able to rebuild in the short term, with 2021 not being the year we will see a return to the economic level before the pandemic.

It is clear that the world has not been and is not prepared for pandemics. We cannot forget that people are not numbers. Each life is important, and pandemics need to be seriously combated with public policies and science. Our leaders need to have a long-term vision in relation to public health and how to solve economic problems with greater agility, because in such crisis, workers' income fall and so does the level of employment and the income of companies, as we saw in this study.

This analysis is still incomplete, as we do not have a vaccine that will put an end to this pandemic. The methods for combating it are palliative, the knowledge of COVID-19 is still minimal, and even today, as yesterday, measures such as social distance and wearing masks can protect us from contagion. The number of vaccines under development in various parts of the world as of July 2020 was 166, with at least 24 of them being tested on humans, according to the WHO. The tests of four vaccines involved the participation of Brazil. Five of these were already in Phase 3: the one developed by Sinovac (China), the one by Sinopharm with the Wuhan Biological Institute (China), Sinopharm in partnership with the Beijing Biological Institute (China), the one developed by the University of Oxford (United Kingdom), and the one by Modena (United States). Of these, two (Sinovac and Oxford) are conducting tests in Brazil.

References

1. Atlas Histórico do Brasil - Fundação Getúlio Vargas (FGV). Retrieved from: https://atlas.fgv.br/verbetes/gripe-espanhola (accessed on July 27, 2020).
2. Bertucci-Martins, L. M. (2003). "Conselhos ao povo": educação contra a influenza de 1918, *Cadernos Cedes*, **23**(59), pp. 103–118.
3. Bresser-Pereira, L. C., et al. (2017). *Macroeconomia desenvolvimentista: teoria e política do novo-desenvolvimentismo*. São Paulo: GEN Atlas.
4. Christensen, T., et al. (2016). Comparing coordination structures for crisis management in six countries, *Public Administration*, **94**(2), pp. 316–332.
5. Correia, S., Luck, S. and Verner, E. (2020). Pandemics depress the economy, public health interventions do not: evidence from the 1918 Flu. Retrieved from: https://papers.ssrn.com/sol3/DisplayJournalBrowse.cfm (accessed on July 03, 2020).
6. Croda, J. H. R. and Garcia, L. P. (2020). Resposta imediata da Vigilância em Saúde à epidemia da COVID-19, *Epidemiologia e Serviços de Saúde*, **29**(1), p. e2020002.
7. De Matos, H. J. (2018). A próxima pandemia: estamos preparados?, *Revista Pan-Amazônica de Saúde*, **9**(3), p. 3.
8. Keynes, J. M. (1964). *The General Theory of Employment, Interest and Money*. New York: Harcourt Brace.
9. Werneck, G. L. and Carvalho, M. S. (2020). A pandemia de COVID-19 no Brasil: crônica de uma crise sanitária anunciada, *Cadernos de Saúde Pública* [online]. **36**(5). Retrieved from: <https://doi.org/10.1590/0102-311X00068820>. ISSN 1678-4464. https://doi.org/10.1590/0102-311X00068820 (accessed on August 08, 2020).
10. Estado de Minas – International (2018). Cem anos depois, Gripe Espanhola carrega lições a próxima pandemia. Retrieved from: https://www.em.com.br/app/noticia/internacional/2018/10/08/ interna_internacional,995639/cem-anos-depois-gripe-espanhola-carrega-licoes-para-a-proxima-pandemi.shtml (accessed on July 03, 2020).
11. Fiocruz, Fundação Osvaldo Cruz, Impactos sociais, econômicos, culturais e políticos da pandemia. Retrieved from: https://portal.fiocruz.br/impactos-sociais-economicos-culturais-e-politicos-da-pandemia (accessed on July 13, 2020).

12. Politize, Gripe Espanhola: a Grande pandemia do século XX. Retrieved from https://www.politize.com.br/gripe-espanhola/ (accessed on July 05, 2020).

13. Revista de pesquisa FAPES: a espera da pandemia - Rodrigo de Oliveira Andrade, abr. 2018 ed. 266. Retrieved from: https://revistapesquisa.fapesp.br/senhora-do-caos/ (accessed on July 04, 2020).

Chapter 10

New Legalization for COVID-19

Márcio Teixeira Bittencourt,[a] Germana Menescal Bittencourt,[b] and Katiucia Nascimento Adam[b]

[a] Pará Court of Justice and Federal University of Pará, Av. Almirante Barroso, 3089, Belém, Pará 66.613-710, Brazil
[b] Federal University of Pará, Rua Augusto Correa, 01 Belém, Pará 66.075-110, Brazil
marciobitten@gmail.com, germana.menescal@gmail.com, katiucia@ufpa.br

This chapter deals with the description and analysis of the legislation that came into force in Brazil as a result of the COVID-19 pandemic. As an approach, emphasis will be placed on analysis of the effectiveness of public environmental and sanitary control policies and access to sanitation. Methodically, we will start from the joint responsibility of the federal, state, and municipal federated entities set out in Theme 793 of the Brazilian Federal Supreme Court in relation to health care. With the application of Federal Law N° 13,979/2020, after the judgment of the Direct Action of Unconstitutionality (ADI) 6341, in April 2020, Article 3 shall be interpreted according to the Federal Constitution for the purpose of determining how each of the federated entities may legislate on COVID-19 and the implementation of restrictive measures of sanitary control and facing the public health emergency. Structurally, a topic will be dedicated to the relaxation of environmental

Living with COVID-19: Economics, Ethics, and Environmental Issues
Edited by Chaudhery Mustansar Hussain and Gustavo Marques da Costa
Copyright © 2022 Jenny Stanford Publishing Pte. Ltd.
ISBN 978-981-4877-78-7 (Hardcover), 978-1-003-16828-7 (eBook)
www.jennystanford.com

legislation during the COVID-19 pandemic and the consequences on environmental degradation; one topic will be on health control aspects, with lockdown decrees and the mandatory use of protective masks; and one topic will be on the new sanitation regulatory framework established by Law N° 14,026/2020 and the positive and negative aspects in relation to COVID-19. The case study will include the territorial outline of the Metropolitan Region of Belém-PA and will analyze the effectiveness and divergences of the COVID-19 legislation in relation to the Federal Union, the State of Pará, and the municipality of Belém.

10.1 Universal Access to Health in Brazil and the Responsibility of the Federated Entities

The main focus for contemplating health control and the legislation of COVID-19 in Brazil starts from the great differential of access to the Universal Health System, enshrined in the Constitution of the Republic in its Article 196, which expressly states that access to health is a right of all and a duty of the state that it must guarantee through social and economic policies aimed at reducing the risk of disease and other aggravations and universal and equal access to actions and services for its promotion, protection, and recovery. Article 200 provided for the creation of the Unified Health System (SUS, Brasil, 1990). Thus, if access to health is a universal right in Brazil, necessarily so is access to public health control policies related to the COVID-19 pandemic.

The materialization of universal access to health occurs through the SUS, created by Federal Law N° 8,080/90, stipulating in Article 2 that health is a fundamental human right and the state must provide the necessary conditions for its full exercise (Brasil, 1990).

Since access control to health control is universal, it is due to the government public environmental policies, health control, and access to sanitation with an emphasis on prevention, protection, and recovery of citizens in general, regarding to the COVID-19 pandemic. On February 3, 2020, the Brazilian Ministry of Health published Ordinance N° 188/2020, declared a Public Health Emergency of

National Importance (ESPIN in Portuguese) due to the human infection with the new coronavirus SARS-CoV-2 (BRASIL, 2020a).

Within the parameters of the Democratic State of Law in which the federative pact is stablished with the sharing of powers and respective responsibilities among the federated entities, the great challenge is a joint action among the union, the 26 states, the Federal District, including the 5570 municipalities emphasizing that the public health control policies related to the COVID-19 pandemic need to include more than 210 million inhabitants (Instituto Brasileiro de Geografia e Estatística [IBGE], 2020).

Even though it is consolidated among the superior courts that the responsibility in relation to health care is jointly held among the federated entities of the union, that is, states, Federal District, and municipalities, which was established in Theme 793 of the Supreme Federal Court (STF in Brazil), doubts still remain regarding how it will work and how responsibility will be exercised by each of the federative entities. The situation becomes even more complex with regard to the financial resources to cover the respective expenses.

Thus, the Federal Supreme Court, in a decision of general repercussion, fixed the following docket in relation to Theme 793, regarding responsibility in terms of health:

> THEME 793: The federation entities, as a result of common competence, are jointly responsible for the provision of health care, and in view of the constitutional criteria for decentralization and hierarchization, it is due to the judicial authority to direct its compliance, in accordance with the rules of division of competences and determine the reimbursement to those who supported the financial burden (RE 855.178, Rapporteur, Minister Luiz Fux, Editor for the judgment, Minister Edson Fachin, judged in the On-site Plenary on May 23, 2019) (STF, 2019).

For a given subject to be the object of general repercussion, the subject in dispute is a massive and repetitive demand. In other words, even before the COVID-19 pandemic began, the federal entities did not understand each other in terms of the effective exercise of joint responsibility in health care, which is why the decision was embargoed and the referred appeal was analyzed in

April, 2020, when the pandemic was already underway. However, it was limited to establishing that in the case of use of drugs without registration with the National Health Surveillance Agency (ANVISA in Portuguese), actions must necessarily be proposed against the union (STF, 2020).

For example, the interpretation of the judgment in the context of the COVID-19 pandemic is that various types of tests for diagnostic purposes, several drugs (including experimental), and even vaccines are under development but are not authorized by the ANVISA, in which case, if they are used, legal action must be brought against the union.

Solidary responsibility for implementation in relation to public environmental and sanitary control policies, especially with regard to access to the sanitation system and drinking water, is not yet a positive reality to be celebrated.

The Metropolitan Region of Belém (RMB in Portuguese), State of Pará, was chosen as a territorial section for the case study of this chapter. According to the Brazilian Institute of Geography and Statistics (IBGE), the estimated population for the year 2019 in the State of Pará was 8,602,865 inhabitants, occupying the 24th position among the 27 federation units, with a Human Development Index of 0.646. In territorial extension, the State of Pará is the second most extensive, totaling 1,245,759,305 km^2 (IBGE, 2020).

10.2 The Federal Law N° 13,979/2020 and the Competencies to Legislate about COVID-19

In Federal Law N° 13,979/2020, after the judgment of ADI 6341, in April 2020, Article 3 shall be interpreted in accordance with the Federal Constitution in order to determine how each of the federated entities may legislate on COVID-19 and the implementation of restrictive measures of sanitary control and coping with the emergency of public health.

The referred law had its constitutionality questioned before the Federal Supreme Court, exactly with regard to the definition of jurisdiction. The following is a transcription of the summary of the res judicata:

ADI 6341/DF, rapporteur Minister Marco Aurélio – ADI filed against provisions of Law N° 13,979/2020 (items I, II, and VI and §§ 8, 9, 10, and 11 of Article 3), considering chances promoted by Provisional Measure N° 929, of March 20, 2020, which dealt with "isolation, quarantine and mobility restrictions (article 3, I, II e VI) and interdiction of public services and essential activities (article 3, § 8) and the movement of people and cargo (art. 3, § 11), as well as how and who can determine them (art. 3, §§ 8 to 10)." It is argued that (i) the matter requires a complementary law and not a provisional measure and (ii) an offense against federal autonomy (CF, Article 18), to the argument that the rules that were fought would have removed part of the common administrative competence of the states, the Federal District and the municipalities, to adopt, without the participation of the union, isolation measures; quarantine; restriction of locomotion by highways, ports, and airports; and interdiction of essential activities and services, centralizing these measures in the "Presidency of Republic" and in "regulatory agency or the granting or authorizing power" (STF, 2020).

In the preliminary judgment of ADI 6341/DF, it maintained the competencies of the states and municipalities to legislate on COVID-19 under the understanding that it is a common competence. Emphasizing that the offense against administrative autonomy occurred, in particular, due to the fact that the union established the requirements to be fulfilled by the federated entities, as if centralized in the Presidency of the Republic, but without determining where the financial resources would come from.

The court, by majority, endorsed the act, plus interpretation in accordance with the constitution to § 9 of Article 3 of Law N° 13,979/2020, explaining the competence of the President of the Republic to dispose, by decree, on public services and essential activities, preserving the attribution of each entity of the federation.

Federal Law N° 13,979/2020 was regulated by Federal Decree N° 10,2828, on February 6, 2020. The referred decree regulating public services and essential activities practically deflated and made lockdown impossible by greatly expanding the concept of essential activities, leading to the necessity of publishing Federal Decree N° 10,329, on April 28, 2020 (BRASIL, 2020b).

The Ministry of Health Ordinance N° 356/2020, published on March 11, 2020, was limited to dealing with social isolation and quarantine of people infected with coronavirus (COVID-19).

However, Ordinance N° 1,565, of June 18, 2020, of the Ministry of Health, which establishes general guidelines aimed at preventing, controlling, and mitigating the transmission of COVID-19 and promoting the physical and mental health of the Brazilian population in order to contribute to actions for the safe resumption of activities and safe social interaction, expressly provided in the single paragraph of Article 1 on the general guidelines, in order to contribute with actions for the safe resumption of activities and safe social life, in the local sphere.

> Single Paragraph. It is up to the local authorities and local health agencies to decide, after evaluating the epidemiological scenario and the response capacity of health care system, regarding the resumption of activities (BRASIL, 2020c).

How each entity of the federation legislated on the enactment of lockdown and the use of protective masks, taking into account the union, the State of Pará, and the municipality of Belém, will be discussed next.

10.3 Sanitary Control: Case Study

10.3.1 The Lockdown Declaration and the Mandatory Use of Protective Masks in Brazil

At the federal level, the first in-depth technical concept of what the lockdown would be and its difference in relation to social isolation is not included in the legislation, but according to Epidemiologic Bulletin N° 8, of the Health Surveillance Secretariat – Ministry of Health, published in April 9, 2020 (Ministério da Saúde, 2020):

- Lockdown: It is the highest level of security, and it may be necessary in situations of serious threat to the health system. During a lockdown, all entrances are blocked by security workers and no one is allowed to enter or leave the isolated perimeter. The main objective is to interrupt any activity for a short period of time.

- Expanded social distancing: This is a strategy not limited to specific groups, requiring that all sectors of society remain in residence during the term of the measure's decree by local managers. This measure restricts contact between people as much as possible. Essential services are maintained, with the adoption of more rigorous hygiene procedures and avoiding crowds. Its objective is to reduce the speed of propagation of the virus, aiming to save time to equip health services with the minimum operation conditions—beds, respirators, personal protective equipment, laboratory tests, and human resources.
- Selective social distancing: This is a strategy where only a few groups are isolated, including all symptomatic people and their household contacts, as well as the people that are at the greatest risk of developing the disease or those who may have a more severe condition, such as older adults and people with chronic diseases (diabetes, heart conditions, etc.) or risk conditions, such as obesity and risky pregnancy. People under the age of 60 can move freely, maintaining a conduct of social distancing and hygienic care if they are asymptomatic. It aims to promote a gradual return to work activities safely, avoiding an explosion of cases without the local health system having the time to absorb the impact.

The advantages and disadvantages of adopting these measures are summarized in Table 10.1.

However, there was a mismatch between the strategy adopted by the Ministry of Health, following compliance with the rules suggested by the World Health Organization, which had a technical position in favor of expanded social isolation and lockdown, and the Presidency of the Republic, which argued that isolation should be only selective. This divergence culminated in the dismissal of the Minister of Health Luiz Henrique Mandetta, who held the position at the time.

On May 11, 2020, the National Health Council, and advisory body of the Ministry of Health, published Recommendation N° 036, recommending the implementation throughout the country

Table 10.1 Advantages and disadvantages of social distancing measures

Measures	Advantages	Disadvantages
Lockdown	It is effective in reducing the case curve and gives time for reorganization of the health system in a situation of uncontrolled acceleration of cases and deaths. The countries that implemented it managed to get out of the most critical moment faster.	This has a high economic cost.
Expanded social distancing	It is essential when adopted in a timely manner, in order to avoid an uncontrolled acceleration of the disease, which could lead to a collapse of the health system and would also cause economic loss. This measure is not focused on COVID-19 but can be used in all situations of competition for beds and respirators.	The prolonged maintenance of this strategy can cause significant impacts on the economy, and it is difficult to know when to open.
Selective social distancing (DSS)	When the conditions are guaranteed, the resumption of labor and economic activity is possible, as is the gradual creation of herd immunity in a controlled manner and the reduction of social traumas as a result of social distancing.	Even in a DSS strategy, vulnerable groups will continue to come in contact with asymptomatic or symptomatic infected people, making control more difficult. Countries like the United Kingdom that started to take this measure had to back down in view of the dizzying case acceleration without the support of the system. It becomes reckless without the minimum operating condition.

Source: Ministério da Saúde, 2020.

of more restrictive social distancing measures (lockdown) in the municipalities with accelerated occurrence of new cases of COVID-19 and whose services occupancy rate had reached critical levels.

One of the justifications for the recommendation was to contain the uncontrolled advance of the COVID-19 contagion when the measures of social distancing were not having the desired effect, in order to allow the health system to recover and be able to absorb, in the best possible way, the demand, thus making it necessary to completely suspend nonessential activities with restricted movement of people—a measure known as lockdown.

The recommendation was drawn up on the basis of studies developed by different academic institutions, such as the Institute of Studies for Health Policies and the National School of Public Health Sérgio Arouca of the Oswaldo Cruz Foundation (ENSP/Fiocruz), which indicated that the SUS would not have sufficient capacity to care for COVID-19 patients who would require intensive care.

The National Health Council effectively recommended the following measures, within the scope of the Ministry of Health, states and Federal District governors, state health secretaries, municipal mayors, and municipal health secretaries:

- Suspension of all activities not essential to the maintenance of life and health, only authorizing the operation of services considered essential by their nature
- Adoption of guidance and administrative sanction measures when there is a violation of social restriction measures, which can be applied in specific areas of a city (neighborhood, districts, sectors)
- Restriction of the circulation of people and private vehicles (only with the use of protective masks), except for the public transportation of people in the itinerary and in the performance of services considered essential, with expansion of information and educational measures (monitoring of compliance) in vehicles of collective transport
- Mobilization of the armed and security forces, by the state and municipal powers, through intersectoral partnerships between the agencies, in order to comply with the emergency protocols for the adoption of total lockdown when necessary,

with planning prior to the limit of occupancy of beds in the local health system

Thus, the Brazilian federal legislation did not expressly contemplate the lockdown, being limited to dealing with social isolation, quarantine, and other restrictive measures. Likewise, the use of protective masks has never been mandatory, being limited to the recommendation to use, through Ordinance N° 1,565, of June 18, 2020, of the Ministry of Health.

10.3.2 Lockdown Decree and Use of Protective Masks in the State of Pará

In the State of Pará, State Decree N° 609, of March 16, 2020, which represents a milestone in restrictive measures to control the COVID-19 pandemic (Pará, 2020a), presented as a territorial scope all 144 municipalities that make up the State of Pará. However, it did not decree lockdown measures.

It contemplated home isolation of at least 14 days for all who entered the territory (Article 7), including penalty of civil, administrative, and penal liability of the offending agent, under the terms of Interministerial Ordinance N° 5, of March 17, 2020.

Regarding the use of protective masks, State Decree N° 609, of March 16, 2020, made specific regulation, until May 15, 2020, as consolidated in Table 10.2.

The State of Pará was the second Brazilian state to declare the lockdown. Unlike Maranhão, there was no judicialization, but State Decree N° 729, of May 5, 2020, was published:

> Provides for the total suspension of non-essential activities (lockdown), within the scope of the Municipalities of Belém, Ananindeua, Marituba, Benevides, Castanhal, Santa Isabel do Pará, Santa Bárbara do Pará, Breves, Vigia and Santo Antônio do Tauá, aiming to contain the uncontrolled advance of the COVID-19 Pandemic (Pará, 2020b).

Territorially, in addition to the municipalities that make up the RMB (Belém, Ananindeua, Marituba, Benevides, Castanhal, Santa Isabel do Pará, Santa Bárbara do Pará), a lockdown was decreed in

Table 10.2 Regulation of the use of protective masks in the State of Pará

Legal provision	Nature	Mask use
Article 8	Passenger transport, public or private	Do not allow people without masks to enter the vehicles.
Article 11, item III and single paragraph	Banking, public and private	Prevent access to the establishment of people without masks.
Article 16, item I	Presential cults and religious events—prohibited	Allow the meeting of maximum 10 persons, with mandatory use of masks.
Article 16, item III	Bus stops	Make use of masks mandatory.
Article 21	Engineering worksite	Ensure supply of masks to workers.
Article 22	Commercial establishments	Prevent access to the establishment of people without a mask.

Source: Pará, 2020a.

three municipalities in the interior of the state—the municipality of Breves, located on Marajó Island, and the municipalities of Vigia and Santo Antônio do Tauá, located in the Salgado Paraense region.

The normative lockdown instrument had a predetermined term, that is, it started on May 7, 2020, and ended on May 17, 2020. It brought expressly in §1 of Article 2 the mandatory use of protective masks. In other words, in the permitted cases of movement of people, the use of a mask was mandatory.

Considering the continuity of the uncontrolled advance of the COVID-19 pandemic, on May 16, 2020, through the publication in Official Gazette N° 34,220, temporary measures for total suspension of nonessential activities (lockdown) were extended to cover seven more municipalities: Cametá, Canaã dos Carajás, Parauapebas, Marabá, Santarém, Abaetetuba, and Capanema. The term was also extended to include the period from May 19, 2020, to May 24, 2020, while the use of protective masks in exceptional cases of movement of persons remained mandatory (Pará, 2020c).

On May 24, 2020, State Decree N° 777/2020 was published, related to restrictions on the movement of people after lockdown

Table 10.3   Classification of zones by risk levels (flags)

	Zone	Flag	Risk level
1	Zone 00: Lockdown	Black	Lockdown
2	Zone 01: Maximum alert	Red	High risk
3	Zone 02: Control I	Orange	Medium risk
4	Zone 03: Control II	Yellow	Intermediate risk
5	Zone 04: Partial opening	Green	Low risk
6	Zone 05: New normal	Blue	Minimum risk

Source: Pará, 2020e.

(Pará, 2020d). This decree provides for the measures of controlled distancing, aiming at preventing and facing the pandemic of COVID-19, within the scope of the State of Pará, and revokes State Decree N° 609, of March 20, 2020. However, 1 week later, it was also revoked by State Decree N° 800/2020, of May 31, 2020 (Pará, 2020e).

State Decree N° 800/2020 instituted the RETOMAPARÁ project, providing for the safe economic and social resumption, within the scope of the State of Pará, through the application of controlled distancing measures and specific protocols for the gradual reopening and operation of segments of both activities, economic and social, and revoked State Decree N° 729, of May 5, 2020, and State Decree N° 777, of May 23, 2020.

Annex II to the aforementioned decree creates a regional division of the state into eight regions, which are now classified by risk level, indicated by colors compatible with the degree of risk, described in Table 10.3.

10.4 New Regulatory Framework for Sanitation in Brazil

The new regulatory framework for basic sanitation in Brazil was established by Law N° 14,026, of July 15, 2020. Some of the main themes dealt with by the new law deal with the universalization of sanitation services and the establishment of a new deadline for the end of dumps in the country.

The need for solutions to be devised for the situation of nonaccess to basic sanitation in Brazil is a reality that is very well portrayed by the research developed by the Trata Brazil Institute. The institute, in partnership with GO Associados, publishes the ranking of basic sanitation of the 100 largest cities in Brazil. The report of 2020 was used as a reference, which includes water and sewage indicators in the largest cities in the country based on data from the National Information System (base year 2018), released annually by the Ministry of Cities (Instituto Trata Brasil, 2020).

According to the ranking, which includes the best and worst rates of treated sewage related to the water consumed, the city of Belém, capital of the State of Pará, appears in the ranking at one of the worst positions (95th position), with only 2.33% coverage. An even worse situation is presented by the municipality of Ananindeua, the second-most-populous municipality in the State of Pará, which also makes up the RMB, occupying the 97th position, with only 1.75% coverage (Instituto Trata Brasil, 2020).

In terms of the rates of urban sewage service also the situations in Belém and Ananindeua are the worst. Belém appears in the 95th position, with only 13.68% coverage. Ananindeua occupies the last position in the ranking, with only 2.06% coverage (Instituto Trata Brasil, 2020).

Other strikingly negative data were presented by researchers and experts, such as the study by the Secretariat for Economic Policy (SPE), which showed that states that invest less in basic sanitation services may show more deaths from COVID-19. The finding made by the SPE (2020) was that the better the provision of basic sanitation services in the country, the lower the chances of deaths from the new coronavirus.

In the RMB, a city mentioned by the SPE study, more than 2 million inhabitants (90.1%) do not have access to sewage collection and more than 900,000 (39.8%) do not receive treated water from the taps of their homes. The study gathered information from the Ministry of Health, IBGE (2020), and Instituto Trata Brasil.

In late April, a study by the Oswaldo Cruz Foundation (Fiocruz) also found genetic material for the new coronavirus inside the sewage system in Niterói (Rio de Janeiro). The locations chosen for sample collection included drainage inlets, treatment stations, and

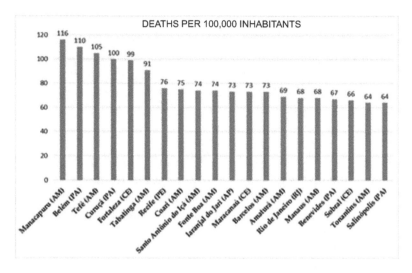

Figure 10.1   Cities with the highest mortality by COVID-19 in Brazil. *Source*: Secretarias de Saúde Estaduais, 2020.

points for the discharge of hospital sewage. In the first published result, traces of the virus were found in 5 of the 12 areas surveyed.

Figure 10.1 shows the 20 cities with the highest mortality from COVID-19, updated on June 10, 2020 by the state health departments. Belém is the second city with the highest mortality in the country, presenting a rate of 110 deaths per 100,000 inhabitants. According to the figure, of the 20 cities with the highest mortality from COVID-19, 18 are located in the north and northeast regions of Brazil, where sanitation rates are the worst.

The figures presented during the COVID-19 pandemic in Brazil made it clear that the worse the sanitation rates, the more serious are the consequences of COVID-19. Therefore, the universalization of sanitation services proposed by the new sanitation framework is so urgent. The law provides that companies must expand the supply of water to 99% of the population and the collection and treatment of sewage to 90% of the population by the end of 2033. But there is the possibility of extending the term to the year 2040 if technical or financial unfeasibility is proven.

However, the solution given for achieving universal sanitation in Brazil is the privatization of services, because of the fact that there is poor management of public utilities and this is the main reason why universalization has not been achieved so far. In fact, there are several studies that prove the inefficiency of the public authorities and the lack of investments in the sector.

However, other questions must be raised. Private companies are more efficient as they target profits and some regions that are difficult to access and occupied by low-income populations, where there is often a need for lower tariffs, may not be seen as good business by these companies. For these cases, the solution provided by law is to regionalize the provision of the service so that companies cannot provide services only to the municipalities of interest to them, only those that are seen as profitable. Regionalized provision includes municipalities that are both more and less economically interesting for the company providing the service. This regionalization is carried out by the states, which must compose the blocks of municipalities that may collectively contract the services.

It is important to remember that some measures taken during the COVID-19 pandemic included the suspension of the cut of basic services, such as water supply and electricity, and this may be considered a negative aspect for private concessionaires.

Another negative aspect of this model is the international experience in privatization of sanitation services, in which the service, after being privatized, returned to the municipality. According to a study by the Transnational Institute (2017), more than 300 cities in 36 countries have remunicipalized their water and sewage treatment services.

10.5 Flexibilizing Environmental Legislation During the COVID-19 Pandemic and the Consequent Environmental Degradation

It is not the intention of this chapter to go deeper into all the normative flexibility measures adopted by the Federal Government with respect to environmental legislation. We will deal only with those considered to be the main ones. However, it is important to point out that the internal regulations of the federal bodies that are part of the National Environment System (Sistema Nacional do Meio Ambiente), responsible for exercising the police power and fiscalization (Brazilian Institute for the Environment and Renewable Natural Resources and the Chico Mendes Institute for Biodiversity Protection), also underwent major changes, always aimed at flexibility. According to official data from the National Institute for Space Research (INPE, 2020):

- Deforestation alerts in the Amazon rainforest grew by 63.75% in April 2020, when compared to the same month of the previous year, according to the Deter-B system, developed by INPE.
- In 2020, alerts were issued for 405.6 km^2, while in the previous year, in the same period, alerts were issued for 247.7 km^2.

In 2019 alone, Brazil went through three major environmental crises involving the exploitation of natural resources: rupture of the dam in Brumadinho (January, 2019); fires in the Amazon Forest (August–September, 2019), and oil spills in the coastal zone (September–October, 2019). The year 2020 started with the biggest global crisis in recent decades, the COVID-19 pandemic (Santos, 2020).

In view of the territorial cut proposal, the statistical data of all judicial units that directly address environmental issues in the municipality of Belém were catalogued. They could be called specialized judicial units in environmental matters, two of which were within the scope of the State Court of Justice (Pará), that is, the Environmental Court of Belém and the 5th Court of the Public Treasury of the Capital (Belém). Within the scope of the Federal Justice, data from the 9th Federal Court of Belém were catalogued, also with specialized competence in environmental matters.

A specific request was prepared in April 2020 for data collection from the Statistics Coordinator of the Pará State Court of Justice. Thus, Figs. 10.2 and 10.3 were prepared on the basis of the Statistical Yearbook of the Pará State Court of Justice, base year of 2018, with information update for the years 2019 and 2020 and data verification by the Statistics Coordinator of the Pará State Court of Justice (TJPA, 2020).

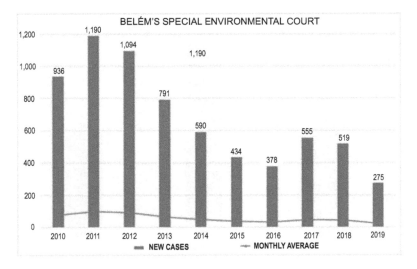

Figure 10.2 New cases filed in Belém's Special Environmental Court. *Source*: TJPA, 2020.

In relation to the data of the 9th Federal Court of Belém, its data came from the Statistical Reporting System Transparency in Numbers, prepared by the Federal Court of Justice – Federal Regional Court of the 1st Region (TRF1, 2020).

The consolidated data showed the number of lawsuits initiated per year with an environmental theme, for the purpose of calculating the monthly average to be compared with the number of actions initiated during the COVID-19 pandemic.

At the Environmental Criminal Court of Belém, the number of cases initiated in 2019 was lower than in the preceding 10 years. When compared to the year of 2018, it practically halved, reaching a monthly average of 23 new cases (Fig. 10.2). Comparatively, the year 2020 shows a considerable decrease in the number of new actions: 49 new actions were filed in January, 23 in February, and only 7 actions in March. After March, the system was no longer fed new information.

Another judicial unit that receives actions related to environmental conflicts and also issues related to health is the 5th Court of the Public Treasury of the Capital (Belém), which has competence for homogeneous, collective, and individual rights. The court was

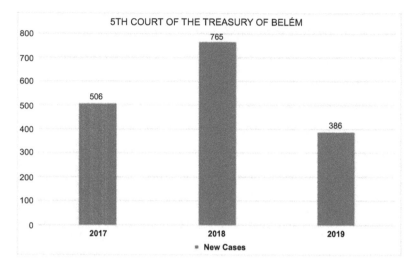

Figure 10.3 New cases in the 5th Court of the Public Treasury of Belém. *Source*: TJPA, 2020.

Table 10.4 New cases filed in the 5th Court of Public Treasury of the Capital (Belém) in 2020

5th Court of Public Treasury of Belém (2020)					
Jan	Feb	Mar	Apr	May	Jun
14	29	15	19	32	30

created by State Law N° 8,099/2015, contemplating actions for damage liability caused to the environment, and started operating in 2017. Figure 10.3 brings the new cases filed in the years 2017–2019.

In 2020, new actions were registered until June, as can be analyzed by the data in Table 10.4. That is, in the first six months of 2020, only 139 new lawsuits were initiated. A comparison of these numbers with those of previous years shows considerable decrease in cases, similarly to what occurred in the Special Environmental Court.

Regarding the 9th Federal Court of Belém, the arithmetic average of the annual distribution in the preceding 10 years was 945 cases initiated per year, reaching the average monthly distribution in the preceding 10 years of 79 processes per month. The average monthly distribution in the first five months of 2020, which includes the COVID-19 pandemic period, was only 32 cases per month, much lower when compared to the preceding three years, which presented monthly averages of 91, 57, and 46 cases for the years of 2017, 2018, and 2019, respectively.

In conclusion, despite the considerable increase in deforested areas, the number of processes with an environmental theme in Belém has decreased considerably in the last two years. In 2020, the decrease was even more abrupt, which is directly related to the decrease in inspection.

10.6 Conclusions

The chapter addressed issues related to legislation that had to be formulated or readjusted during the COVID-19 pandemic in Brazil, analyzed decisions taken at different levels of government, and presented a brief discussion on the new regulatory framework for sanitation in Brazil.

Brazil, due to its continental dimensions and social and political organization, is a country formed by 26 states and a Federal District, with approximately 210 million inhabitants according to the last census. In such a large country, inequalities are also present. Some regions have suffered more from the pandemic effects, and studies have shown that capitals that have the worst sanitation rates and also the highest mortality rates due to COVID-19 in the country.

The country reached the 100,000 COVID-19 death mark on August 8, 2020, five months after the country's first recorded case. Brazil ranks second in the number of deaths in the world and the first in Latin America, adding by itself more deaths than its neighboring countries. There were several factors that contributed to this sad statistic: the lethality of the virus, the delay in some decision making by the public authorities, the impasse between legislation adopted by different states and the union, low rates of sanitation services coverage in some regions of the country, and lack of capacity of the SUS (the largest universal health system in the world) to absorb this kind of emergency.

The universalization of sanitation services is one of the goals of the new regulatory framework that was sanctioned in July 2020, since data from 2018 show that only 83.62% of the population is served by water supply services and 53.15% is served by sewage collection and treatment services in Brazil (Governança, Planejamento e Gestão Estratégica de Serviços Municipais de Água e Esgoto, 2020).

The issue of environmental flexibilization was also addressed, analyzing the cases with environmental themes registered in the courts of Belém, both state and federal courts, comparing the data with those of previous years. It was found that although environmental degradation has increased, enforcement has decreased and it is therefore not possible to legally demand remediation of environmental damage due to a lack of materiality, making visible during the COVID-19 pandemic the flexibilization of environmental legislation.

References

1. Brasil (1990). [Constituição (1988)]. *Constituição da República Federativa do Brasil: promulgada em 5 de outubro de 1988.* 4ª. ed. São Paulo.
2. Brasil (2020a). Ministério da Saúde. Portaria n° 188, de 03 de fevereiro de 2020, publicada no DOU. 4.2.2020. Declara Emergência em Saúde Pública de importância Nacional (ESPIN) em decorrência da Infecção Humana pelo novo Coronavírus (2019-nCoV). Disponível em: http://www4. planalto.gov.br/legislacao/portal-legis/legislacao-covid-19 (acesso em Agosto de 2020).
3. Brasil (2020b). Decreto Federal n° 10.329, 28 de Abril de 2020. Regulamenta e Define os serviços públicos e as atividades essenciais. Disponível em: http://www.planalto.gov.br/ccivil_03/_ato2019-2022/2020/decreto/D10329.htm#art2 (acesso em Agosto de 2020).
4. Brasil (2020c). Ministério da Saúde. Portaria n° 1.565, de 18 de Junho de 2020. Retomada segura das atividades e o convívio social seguro. Disponível em: https://www.in.gov.br/en/web/dou/-/portaria-n-1.565-de-18-de-junho-de-2020-262408151 (acesso em Agosto de 2020).
5. Governança, Planejamento e Gestão Estratégica de Serviços Municipais de Água e Esgoto – GESAE (2020). Sistema CFA – Conselho Federal

de Administração. Disponível em: https://gesae.org.br/mesorregioes (acesso em Agosto de 2020).

6. Instituto Brasileiro de Geografia e Estatística – IBGE (2020). Censo Demográfico 2020. Números do Censo 2020. Disponível em: https://censo2020.ibge.gov.br/sobre/numeros-do-censo.html (acesso em Agosto de 2020).

7. Instituto Nacional de Pesquisas Espaciais – INPE (2020). Disponível em: http://www.obt.inpe.br/OBT/assuntos/programas/amazonia/prodes (acessado em abril de 2020).

8. Instituto Transnacional (2017). Remunicipalización. Como ciudades y ciudadanía están escribiendo el futuro de los servicios públicos. Disponível em: https://cdnstatic8.com/fnucut.org.br/wp-content/uploads/2018/11/Estudo-sobre-remunicipalizacao-dos-servi%C3%A7os-p%C3%BAblicos.pdf (acesso em Agosto de 2020).

9. Instituto Trata Brasil (2020). Ranking do Saneamento de 2020. Sistema Nacional de Informações sobre Saneamento (SNIS) – ano base 2018 - Ministério das Cidades. Disponível em: http://tratabrasil.org.br/estudos/estudos-itb/itb/ranking-do-saneamento-2020 (acesso em Agosto de 2020).

10. Ministério da Saúde (2020). Boletim Epidemiológico n° 8 da Secretaria de Vigilância em Saúde, Ministério da Saúde, publicado em 09 de abril de 2020 - Semana Epidemiológica 15. Ministério da Saúde. Disponível em: https://www.saude.gov.br/images/pdf/2020/April/09/be-covid-08-final.pdf (acesso em Agosto de 2020).

11. Pará (2020a). Decreto Estadual n° 609, de 16 de março de 2020. Dispõe sobre as medidas de enfrentamento, no âmbito do Estado do Pará, à pandemia do COVID-19. Disponível em: https://www.legisweb.com.br/legislacao/?id=391233 (acesso em Agosto de 2020).

12. Pará (2020b). Decreto Estadual n° 729, de 5 de Maio de 2020. Dispõe sobre a suspensão total de atividades não essenciais (lockdown). Disponível em: https://www.sistemas.pa.gov.br/sisleis/legislacao/5578 (acesso em Agosto de 2020).

13. Pará (2020c). Diário Oficial n° 34.220, 16 de maio de 2020. Dispõe sobre a ampliação do lockdown. Disponível em: http://www.pge.pa.gov.br/content/legislacoescovid19 (acesso em Agosto de 2020).

14. Pará (2020d). Decreto Estadual n° 777/2020, publicado no dia 24 de maio de 2020. http://www.pge.pa.gov.br/sites/default/files/de777revogado.pdf. Disponível em: http://www.pge.pa.gov.br/content/legislacoescovid19 (acesso em Agosto de 2020).

15. Pará (2020e). Decreto Estadual n° 800/2020, publicado no dia 31 de maio de 2020. http://www.pge.pa.gov.br/sites/default/files/de777revogado.pdf. Disponível em: http://www.pge.pa.gov.br/content/legislacoescovid19 (acesso em Agosto de 2020).

16. Santos, Boaventura de Sousa. A Cruel Pedagogia do Vírus (2020). Disponível em: https://www.almedina.net/a-cruel-pedagogia-do-v-rus-1586961170.html (acesso em 25 out. 2019).

17. Secretaria de Política Econômica – SPE (2020). Ministério da Economia. Falta de Saneamento Piora o Combate ao Coronavírus. Disponível em: http://cfa.org.br/falta-de-saneamento-piora-o-combate-ao-coronavirus/ (acesso em Agosto de 2020).

18. Secretarias Estaduais de Saúde (2020). Gráfico das cidades com maior incidência de casos de COVID-19. Dados tabulados as 11h50 de 10 de junho. Disponível em: https://g1.globo.com/ap/amapa/noticia/2020/05/26/covid-19-3-municipios-do-amapa-aparecem-entre-as-10-maiores-incidencias-de-casos-do-pais.ghtml (acesso em Agosto de 2020).

19. Supremo Tribunal Federal – STF (2019). Embargos Declaratórios Sob Ação Direta De Inconstitucionalidade ADI 6341 (Decisão de 15/04/2020, publicada no DJe em 07/05/2020). Disponível em: http://www.stf.jus.br/portal/cms/verTexto.asp?servico=resumocovid&pagina=resumocovid_adi (acesso em Agosto de 2020).

20. Supremo Tribunal Federal (2020). Embargos Declaratórios no Recurso Extraordinário 855.178 Sergipe. Embargos de Declaração desp. Publicação: 16/04/2020. Disponível em: http://stf.jus.br/portal/jurisprudenciaRepercussao/verAndamentoProcesso.asp?incidente=4678356&numeroProcesso=855178&classeProcesso=RE&numeroTema=793 (acesso em Agosto de 2020).

21. Tribunal de Justiça do Estado do Pará. Anuário Estatístico (2020). Disponível em: http://www.tjpa.jus.br/PortalExterno/hotsite/anuario-estatistico-2018/ (acesso em abril de 2020).

22. Tribunal Regional Federal da 1ª Região – TRF1 (2020). Sistema de Relatórios Estatísticos Transparência em Números, elaborado pelo Conselho de Justiça Federal. Disponível em: https://portal.trf1.jus.br/portaltrf1/transparencia/estatisticas-processuais/ (acesso em Agosto de 2020).

Chapter 11

Modern Policy and Decision Making about COVID-19

Wilson Engelmann,[a] Jéferson Alexandre Rodrigues,[a] and Haide Maria Hupffer[c]

[a]*UNISINOS, Unisinos Avenue 950, 93022-750, São Leopoldo, Rio Grande do Sul, Brazil*
[b]*Feevale University, ERS-239, 2755, 93525-075, Novo Hamburgo, Rio Grande do Sul, Brazil*
wengelmann@unisinos.br, roodrigues.adv@gmail.com, haide@feevale.br

The twenty-first century will be remembered not only for the great climatic, social, and political tragedies or advances in science but also for having experienced one of the biggest public health crises ever recorded, COVID-19. The pandemic brought with it a series of questions that forced world leaders to have immediate and plausible answers in order to mitigate the effects generated by the new corona virus. However, from a quick analysis of the measures taken by government officials (not in the majority) what is envisaged are numerous actions based on more uncertainties generated than really effective responses. The disagreement between guidelines and means of mitigating the effects of the pandemic, even after months of its enactment by the WHO, still reflects the neglect and the lack of preparedness of humanity to cross something like this. Through Ulrich Beck's *Metamorphosis of the World*, we will bring concepts and reflexes related to the pandemic, which are nothing more than

Living with COVID-19: Economics, Ethics, and Environmental Issues
Edited by Chaudhery Mustansar Hussain and Gustavo Marques da Costa
Copyright © 2022 Jenny Stanford Publishing Pte. Ltd.
ISBN 978-981-4877-78-7 (Hardcover), 978-1-003-16828-7 (eBook)
www.jennystanford.com

the obsolete and plastered form that society and law are seen. It is necessary to reflect on the law on the basis of this new social bias, linked to globalization and the Fourth Industrial Revolution.

11.1 Introduction

This century, throughout its initial years, was already emerging as a century focused on innovation, development, and scientific advances; hence the scenario of the Fourth Industrial Revolution is outlined. The achievements hitherto only dreamed of by man slowly became a reality because if before they were created in the field of utopia, today they are produced and commercialized in the factual world. However, something that escaped even the most distant propositions of man happened, something that for this century was not on the agenda: the pandemic by the new coronavirus—COVID-19.

The pandemic caused by the new coronavirus came as a watershed, since it exacerbated public health crises already existing around the globe, bringing the need for support both in the field of medicine (in order to have a quick and effective answer about the dimension of the problem) and regulatory analysis in order to safeguard rights and duties that end up being overshadowed, due to the infamous "collective good at the expense of the individual."

In this sense, there is the idea of *Metamorphosis of the World*, taught by Beck [4], which is based exactly on the epicenter of the problem brought by COVID-19: decision-making. From a social point of view, for example, numerous uncertainties emerge when there is a pandemic, as the proposal for social distance adopted by much of the world was not well received by the population or even respected. Depending on Beck's theory [4], the pandemic brought about a significant change in worldviews in a global context.

This chapter will aim to work on the idea of Beck's *Metamorphosis of the World* [4], incorporating it into the reality brought by the new coronavirus. The aim will be to analyze how the law should position itself in the face of so many uncertainties that arise from decision-making that theoretically would be destined to reduce the impacts suffered by the pandemic. The intention is not to exhaustively address the problem proposed above but, rather, to plant the seed of doubt about the frequent questions that we are obliged to answer due to this global, noncosmopolitan society.

11.2 COVID-19 Pandemic: Prelude, Reflexes, and Consequences

Saying that you are facing a pandemic is different from saying that you are experiencing a local epidemic. The virus itself, which is currently new, is linked to some disease, changing and appearing in a point on the planet. After this mutation, it spreads along trade routes and travel routes to other parts of the world. Tourists and business travelers have historically been the main carriers of viruses around the globe. When talking about transmission on commercial routes, it is no longer possible to outline a geographically continuous pattern; on the contrary, a disease/virus spreads along these routes from one shopping center to another, crossing the borders of nation-states. Faced with this scenario, widespread and almost simultaneous surges result worldwide, which can, in turn, lead to a later transmission. Here we are facing the first phase of a pandemic [8].

Brazil, like all countries across the globe, is experiencing one of its biggest health crises ever recorded; it can be said that the Spanish flu played out in very similar proportions; however, a different factor in the equation of this pandemic makes it difficult to rule out globalization. Due to the contours brought by the Fourth Industrial Revolution, the risks today can no longer be seen only from the perspective of territoriality and temporality, but, rather, by the ruptures of space and time that scientific and technological advancement provides.

According to data extracted from the Ministry of Health website, Brazil accounted for a total of 116,580 deaths and 3,669,995 infected by COVID-19 as of August 2020. It is important to note that Brazil, since the beginning of the pandemic, has been quite reluctant to adhere to the World Health Organization's (WHO's) recommendations, which possibly holds an intrinsic link to the figures mentioned above [18].

In the Brazilian context, it is possible to analyze an even more complex context, since state governments diverge and introduce, in an autonomous way, different ways of dealing with the pandemic, from meeting the recommendations of the WHO to ignoring them completely. This occurs as a consequence also of the way in which the Federal Government, specifically the President of the Republic, Jair Bolsonaro, places himself above of social reality, where he minimizes the effects generated by COVID-19, even calling it a "small cold" [19].

As mentioned above, one of the major impasses faced over answers about the controversies brought about by COVID-19 was how much each nation was prepared to face the challenges arising from a pandemic. This alleged is seen as a way of preparing for epidemics of infectious diseases in order to reduce their impact on public health. However, what is seen in the current scenario is actually a major failure in this preparation, resulting in health consequences at a global level [19].

It is incontrovertible that pandemics have been experienced throughout human history, causing destructions and social disruptions. However, it is necessary to reflect on what we have learned over the centuries from such ruptures. What did social history teach us? We continue with the same practical short-term actions: although the whole apparatus of the Fourth Industrial Revolution (nanotechnologies, artificial intelligence, robotics, etc.) is available, humanity is conditioned to secular security devices: quarantine, social detachment, closing of state borders, etc. [13].

Health authorities recommend preventive measures, such as washing hands; maintaining social isolation; avoiding touching eyes, nose, and mouth; maintaining respiratory hygiene; using a mask; and seeking medical care. However, a study carried out in Japan pointed out that only the adoption of some preventive measures is insufficient to contain the proliferation. In this regard, the procedures that are available are quarantine, isolation, social detachment, and community containment in order to separate people to interrupt transmission [11].

Notwithstanding these obstacles evidenced by the pandemic, there is an even greater impediment: information—a tsunami of information from everywhere, from scientific research to fanciful ideas covered with supposed truths. Here, it is also possible to cover the extent of the importance of the media and social media (the Fourth Industrial Revolution—emerging technologies), where, with the help of globalization, information that is often wrong can be polarized and reach all corners of the globe, making it even more difficult to work in a pandemic scenario [6]. According to the words of the philosopher Luciano Floridi "information lacks a philosophy, as it must have a semantic character based on data, meaningful and true, where there must be a synergy between knowledge and the information itself" [12, 24].

COVID-19 has also forced us to reflect on the importance of sanitarians—they built the Unified Health System in the last century and through the 1988 Federal Constitution, they made health a universal right and a duty of the state toward the citizen. However, the scrapping of this distribution was even more evident due to the situations experienced by the new coronavirus, which showed the gap between the supplementary medicine offered by the government and the cutting-edge medicine offered by health plans. The paradigm of public health being incorporated into the Federal Constitution came as a means of reiterating the need to safeguard human rights and a right to basic good health [17, 25].

In a scenario ripe with the uncertainty and ignorance brought about by the pandemic, it is necessary to ask the following questions:

- Do not these theoretical uncertainties lead us directly to practical uncertainties on how to deal with the reflexes of the pandemic?
- Understanding the risks inherent in a pandemic, are they the same risks as conceived by classical doctrine?
- How does the pursuit of exacerbated modernization contribute to reaching a state of global health crisis? [26]

The social production of wealth is systematically accompanied by the social production of risk. Such an argument proves to be quite assertive when in the wake of the productive forces, exponentially increasing in the modernization process, risks and potential threats are unleashed/created in a measure hitherto totally unknown, because when it comes to the globalization process, territoriality it is just an innocuous word to measure spaces (strongly what has been seen with the coronavirus, from Asia, but that has spread to all continents) [5].

The impacts suffered by humanity due to the pandemic cannot yet be measured, considering that we are talking about situations that propagate in time or even those that were only enhanced now due to COVID-19 [26]. In addition to the economic scenario, one of the biggest concerns of nonstates is the mental health of people in the face of social isolation and quarantine. We will have instances of morbid people whose condition ended up worsening at home and people who were already sedentary long before the pandemic but whose situation, with social distance, became even worse. We may be talking about an outbreak due to this mental instability, which is often the trigger for many people to stop adhering to the indications of their countries. In other words, a spread of psychopathology can reduce this population's adherence to what we have as preventive measures [2].

At the beginning of the pandemic, one of the biggest concerns of the Chinese era with the mental health of citizens. We thought about how to develop and implement the scope of coverage to alleviate the psychological suffering generated by COVID-19. Through public policies, local authorities were required to incorporate psychological crisis interventions in their training in order to serve the population, so that there were more effective responses to this type of situation [23].

Another serious consequence of social isolation is the leap in the number of cases of domestic violence. Several new problems have also arisen, including physical and psychological health risks, triggering a process of isolation and loneliness because of the closure of many schools and businesses, economic vulnerability, and job losses. It is important to note that the concept of domestic violence here refers to a series of violations that occur within a domestic space [15].

An article published by *The Guardian* referred to the extent to which domestic violence is a behavior repeated throughout the world. An example is an increase of around 40% to 50% in Brazil. In one location in Spain, the government said calls to its helpline increased by 20% in the first days of the confinement period [22]. In the United Kingdom, one of the leading associations helping to prevent domestic violence reported that calls to the UK Domestic Violence Helpline increased by 25% in the seven days after the government's announcement of stricter social detachment. During the same period, there was a 150% increase in visits to the website [3].

11.3 *The Metamorphosis of the World*: Globalization of Risks in the Face of the Pandemic

The Metamorphosis of the World, a work developed by Beck [4], has as its final analysis an observation about the global events that unfold in a society characterized by the disruption of basic concepts that support it. In other words, Beck's theory works synergistically in the context of the pandemic brought about by COVID-19, since these social structures within the context of society are increasingly fragile.

When working on the term "metamorphosis" from the perspective of society, the question arises as to why not use terms such as "social change or transformation." Transformation is interconnected to a kind of evolution from closed to open, from national to global, from poor to rich. In other words, you evolve to the next "level" to which you are allocated. However, metamorphosis means more than just evolving; it is something extraordinary, a reconfiguration of the worldview—what was COVID-19 in the twenty-first century if not a metamorphosis? It is emphasized that for Beck, this metamorphosis cannot come from wars or violence but from a side effect of successful modernization [4].

Beck works with the perspective and meaning of the term "world" when claiming that it undergoes a metamorphosis. Such a claim often delimits the preaching of catastrophists, because for them, a catastrophic analysis when it comes to metamorphosis seems to be a more consistent assessment. Take the example of a caterpillar, for example, where we know that it will morph into a butterfly, but does the caterpillar have such awareness? In other words, catastrophists are the caterpillars, because it is not the world but rather their worldview that undergoes a metamorphosis. Still, one cannot forget also the optimistic view of progressives, who claim that the world will be saved by evolution, but this assertion is also not correct, because the world is actually undergoing surprising global changes, which are seen on the horizon of metamorphosis [4].

The scenario of the new coronavirus proves to be umbilically linked to Beck's theory, as if there had been a premonition, given that the ideals of world and globalization are going through ruptures, "languishing," as the theorist himself says. The path would be cosmopolized actions, which should be understood from national frameworks; in other words, it is necessary to have a cosmopolitan thinking focused on a global movement strategy, as COVID-19 has made something clear: there is no way to escape the globalized reality [4]!

It is possible to affirm that COVID-19 came not only to highlight the twenty-first century in the historical timeline but also to help to actually reconfigure the existing worldview, so the world would understand that in a globalized society, its risks are indisputably global, due to a modernization process (metamorphosis of the world). In other words, it is extremely important to have this macro worldview, interconnected and globalized [10].

11.4 The Law of the Fourth Industrial Revolution and Decision Making about the Risks

Throughout this chapter, we sought to demonstrate that the pandemic brought about by COVID-19 was practically foreseen in Beck's theory—that the risks today must be seen from the perspective of globalization, just as globalization is the result of the Fourth Industrial Revolution, as this modernization is only possible and viable on the basis of a process of scientific and technological advancement [21, 27]. Finally, it is necessary to understand the role of law in this convergence of data and facts in order to make a decision that seeks to mitigate and remove the greatest number of side effects arising from these responses.

"The Fourth Industrial Revolution" is a term coined by economist Klaus Schwab, where for him, in today's society, there is an ongoing paradigm shift that profoundly changes the way we work, communicate, inform ourselves, etc. Uncertainty proves to be a path of no return for development due to the continuous and systematic adoption of emerging technologies (nanotechnology, biotechnology, artificial intelligence, robotics, etc.—technological convergence). Schwab defends the need for a shared comprehensive and global vision in order to face the challenges that constantly arise (the case being totally opposite in the context of COVID-19) [21, 27, 28].

While Beck tried to formulate the details of the stir around metamorphosis and transformation/evolution, Schwab [21, 27] also explains why the Fourth Industrial Revolution is distinct and not just reflections from the Third Industrial Revolution. Let's see [21, 27]:

- Speed: The current industrial revolution evolves in an exponential and nonlinear way due to a globalized world (in metamorphosis), one that is interconnected, given the many emerging technologies that when used in combination can reach extraordinary achievements.
- Breadth and depth: There is the digital revolution as a basis, and it combines several technologies (technological convergence), which results in paradigmatic changes in the economy, in society, and in individuals. The questions are not just about "what" and "how" we do but about "who" we are.
- Systemic impact: There is involvement between countries, both internally and externally, whether in companies, industries, or societies.

It is not just the idea of the world that undergoes a metamorphosis, according to Beck's teachings, but the world industry, since the introduction of these new technologies in a totally digital environment, either through the Internet of Things, artificial intelligence, or big data itself, brings with it great potential for a profound change in the global scenario. With the advent of the Fourth Industrial Revolution, the industry itself is moving toward a reframing that is increasingly open, connected, and involved with society. These new forms of interrelationship will occur in all social fields and in the most diverse segments [20].

Corroborating the provisions regarding scientific evolution and ruptures, Arango and Montenegro conceptualize:

> The dilemma then, if there is one, basically focuses on how different sectors involved will agree to interact with these technologies and delimit their interaction with human beings, and not on whether it will be possible or not, because it is no longer about science fiction literature, but about a trend that does not have turning back. The above, then, is not the future, it is the present; but it is clear that the future is not going to be the continuation of the past. There is a clear break in the solid line (growth or not) caused by changes in people's behaviors, in the way of interacting in the digitally transformed world, but, above all, by the speed of technological change [1].

Again, the systemic brought by the doctrine flows into the reality of the pandemic because the references brought by Schwab [28] were the means by which the virus managed to spread throughout the world. With this bias, it is possible to enter another core of discussion around COVID-19: how should the law position itself in the face of these controversies, arising from a globalized society, in a technological context and undergoing a metamorphosis?

Faced with the reality of COVID-19, we are surrounded by vague predictions about the duration of this abrupt and violent pandemic. Depending on the changes in the shape and magnitude of the socioeconomic consequences, there are still many uncertainties, but one of the biggest questions is around the post-pandemic world— there will be changes, but how these realities will remain and what exactly will remain is unknown [28]. So, the current crisis proves to be a long and opportune moment for reflection on the changing social world and the theories that we can use to make sense of the events that are unfolding [14].

We mentioned above that the ways in which the world dealt with the pandemic generated by COVID-19 still involve archaic and secular actions. In turn, if the law and its normativity are the regulators of society, how we understand it would not be different, since the "plastered and hard" way we interpret it, only from the law put, creates an abyss between law and society because today's law still legislates over a previous society.

To resolve this controversy, the theory of legal pluralism is presented, which arises from the possibility of creating technical standards in order to overcome this bankruptcy created by a legislative process that is slow and sometimes ineffective. It should be said that legal pluralism will be based on principles, such as the precautionary principle, among others, thus demonstrating this normative synergy with the law system [9].

Here we see law from the perspective of a science or social doctrine and its close relationship with the social, political, and cultural dynamics in which it was immersed. This essay turned to the perspective of breaking the idea of this globalized world and asking: we could not start from the recognition of the plurality of law, and recognizing within it there are several ways to recognize it and bring to the field of the factual world. However, so that we can speak in terms of plurality of the sources of law and the ideal "law," it is necessary to understand a series of questions of an epistemological nature, since it is about understanding the nature of the law, its function and relationship with the social environment, and how it becomes the regulatory and normative basis of society [7].

A concept of legal pluralism aims to overcome this centered and reductionist state on the basis of the connection between legal positivism and natural law. An evolution is needed based on the unique idea of legal positivism, where there is no indivisible coexistence between state power and law. One of the great steps of contemporary Europe regarding legal pluralism was the work developed by Paolo Grossi, a great historian of law, where this critic strongly criticized the reductionist idea of law as the strong last element of law and promoted an objective dimension of law as a social institution, seeing legal pluralism more as a consistent order and close to the social context [16].

By legal pluralism, one should understand the possibility that different normative statements coexist, and with them a plurality of legal systems, that is, legal declarations appropriate for or corresponding to a real world, which responds to a factual social reality. Epistemological reflections on the law must be constantly made by analyzing law as a science and its relationship with social reality. Through links (interdisciplinary), the law must analyze social contexts and try to provide answers to these realities that are constantly changing. It is important to mention that the idea of legal pluralism is not reduced to the acceptance of the possibility of several legal systems but those that are based on principles [7].

11.5 Conclusion

The reality experienced by humanity this past year will certainly remain in the history books; it will not be a year remembered for its splendor but for how much humans, even with all the knowledge of technology, are still hostage to a virus that can be easily eliminated with soap and water. Therefore, we were forced to revisit and reflect on several maxims, both in the social and technological context, which until then were seen as irrefutable. COVID-19 has ultimately force us to ask ourselves the following questions [28]: How long does the idea of nationalism actually offer real solutions to problems seen on the global aegis? Would the answer to a globalized society be nationalist isolation?

In this context, it is possible to verify what happened in the national territory, where total sovereignty was exercised over other nation-states, going against any and all scientific data, resulting in thousands of deaths and countless infections. Brazil today ranks second in terms of the number of deaths from the new coronavirus, behind only its "ally" the United States (governed by a sympathizer with local ideals). In other words, society tries to address new problems with old answers, seeing the social reality and the support of the state always in opposing positions.

As we have worked throughout this essay, the proliferation of COVID-19 is inextricably linked to the context of the Fourth Industrial Revolution and its technologies, since they are still part of an attempt to gradually build a social context where more questions are created than answered. The reflexes inherent to this technological revolution are felt daily, which makes us believe in a post-pandemic global society where it is indisputable that actions, forms, and contexts will change, though it is still not known how and for what [21, 27, 28].

The idea is that the world is doomed to metamorphosize, as society changes daily, which makes us reflect on the fact that even in the twenty-first century, with all the technological apparatus, man had to use the same actions that his ancestors used to try to stop the proliferation of a virus: social isolation and quarantine. The daily risk generation to which man is exposed is incalculable; we don't stop building things, improving games and systems, when we have no idea of the tens of thousands of ways that human action has broken the delicate natural ecological balance.

Finally, we mentioned the beginning of a possible action to try to put all social issues that originate into perspective: legal pluralism. The metamorphosis of the world is an undeniable reality; we understand its need for study and being critical, or we will continue to be at the mercy of these risks that are created from a "unannounced" cosmopolitan society. Themes such as the Fourth Industrial Revolution, a post-pandemic global society, and the metamorphosis of the world will need more and more reflection and criticism from the most diverse areas. The concept of interdisciplinarity is increasingly in vogue, as technology, innovation, society, and the regulatory landscape urgently need to find a way to work in order to avoid an implosion at each point mentioned.

References

1. Arango, D. A. J. and Montenegro, D. I. (2019). De la Inteligencia Artificial al juego de los dioses, *Revista ComHumanitas*, **10**(3), pp. 85–106, 2019. Disponível em: http://www.comhumanitas.org/index.php/comhumanitas/article/view/210>(acesso em 27 ago. 2020).

2. Castro-de-Araujo, L. F. S. (2020). Impact of COVID-19 on mental health in a Low and Middle–Income Country, *Ciên. Saúde Colet.*, **25**(1), pp. 2457–2460. Disponível em: https://www.scielo.br/pdf/csc/ v25s1/1413-8123-csc-25-s1-2457.pdf>(acesso em 26 ago. 2020).

3. BBC (2020). Coronavirus: domestic abuse calls up 25% since lockdown, charity says. Disponível em: https://www.bbc.co.uk/news/uk-52157620>(acesso em 27 ago. 2020).

4. Beck, U. (2018). *A Metamorfose do Mundo: Novos Conceitos Para Uma Nova Realidade*, 1st ed. Rio de Janeiro: Zahar.

5. Beck, U. (2011). *Sociedade de Risco: Rumo a Uma Outra Modernidade*, 1st ed. São Paulo: Editora 34.

6. Camargo Jr., K. R. and Goeli, C. M. (2020). A difícil tarefa de informar em meio a uma pandemia, *Phys. Rev. Saúde Colet.*, **30**(2). Disponível em: https://scielosp.org/pdf/physis/2020.v30n2/e300203/pt>(acesso em 25 ago. 2020).

7. Castañeda, C. A. R., Wong, E. M. and Posada, G. J. (2020). Legal pluralism: implications epistemological, *Rev. Derecho del Estado*, **15**, pp. 27–40. Disponível em: https://revistas.ugca.edu.co/index.php/inciso/article/view/71/252>(acesso em 27 ago. 2020).

8. Davies, S. (2020). Pandemics and the consequences of COVID-19, *Econ. Affairs*, **40**(2), pp. 131–137. Disponível em: https://onlinelibrary-wiley.ez101.periodicos.capes.gov.br/doi/full/10.1111/ecaf.12415> (acesso em 27 ago. 2020).

9. Engelmann, W. and Martins, P. S. (2017). A ISO, suas normas e estruturação: possíveis interfaces regulatórias. In: Engelmann, W. and Martins, P. S. (Orgs.) *As Normas ISO e as Nanotecnologias*: entre a autorregulação e o pluralismo jurídico, Karywa, São Leopoldo, pp. 221–227.

10. Ferreira, H. S. and Serraglio, D. A. (2018). Resenha: "a metamorfose do mundo: novos conceitos para uma nova realidade," de Ulrich Beck, *Revista de Direito Econômico e Socioambiental*, **9**(3). Disponível em: https://periodicos.pucpr.br/index.php/direitoeconomico/article/view/24815> (acesso em 25 ago. 2020).

11. Ficanha, E. E., Silva, E. V. da, Rocha, V. M. P., et al. (2020). Aspectos biopsicossociais relacionados ao isolamento social durante a pandemia de COVID-19: uma revisão integrativa. *Res. Soc. Dev.*, **9**(8). Disponível em: https://rsdjournal.org/index.php/rsd/article/view/6410/5868> (acesso em 27 ago. 2020).

12. Floridi, L. (2011). *The Philosophy of Information*. Oxford University. NY: New York.

13. Grisotti, M. (2020). Pandemia de COVID-19: agenda de pesquisas em contexto de incertezas e contribuições das ciências sociais, *Phys. Rev. Saúde Colet.*, **30**(02). Disponível em: https://www.scielo.br/scielo.php?pid=S0103-73312020000200301&script=sci_arttext> (acesso em 25 ago. 2020).

14. Hwang, H. and Höllerer, M. A. (2020). The COVID-19 crisis and its consequences: ruptures and transformations in the global institutional fabric, *J. Appl. Behav. Sci.*, **56**(3), pp. 294–300, 2020. Disponível

em: https://journals-sagepub-com.ez101.periodicos.capes.gov.br/doi/full/10.1177/0021886320936841> (acesso em 27 ago. 2020).

15. Jones, C. B. (2020). The pandemic paradox: The consequences of COVID-19 on domestic violence, *J. Clin. Nurs.*, **29**. Disponível em: https://onlinelibrary-wiley.ez101.periodicos.capes.gov.br/doi/full/10.1111/jocn.15296>(acesso em 27 ago. 2020).

16. Locchi, M. C. (2014). Brief reflections on legal pluralism as a key paradigm of contemporary law in highly differentiated western societies, *Rev. Bras. Direito*, **10**(2), pp. 74–84. Disponível: https://seer.imed.edu.br/index.php/revistadedireito/article/view/635/544> (acesso em 27 ago. 2020).

17. Loyola, M. A. (2020). Basta! Reflexões em torno da COVID-19, *Phys. Rev. Saúde Colet.*, **30**(02). Disponível em: https://www.scielo.br/scielo.php?pid=S0103-73312020000200312&script=sci_arttext> (acesso em 25 ago. 2020).

18. Ministério da Saúde, MS (2020). COVID-19. Disponível em: https://covid.saude.gov.br (acesso em 26 Agosto 2020).

19. Ortega, F. and Behague, D. P. (2020). O que a medicina social latino-americana pode contribuir para os debates globais sobre as políticas da COVID-19: lições do Brasil, *Phys. Rev. Saúde Colet.*, **30**(02). Disponível em: https://www.researchgate.net/publication/342496984_O_que_a_medicina_social_latinoamericana_pode_contribuir_para_os_debates_globais_sobre_as_politicas_da_Covid-19_licoes_do_Brasil>(acesso em 25 ago. 2020).

20. Porath, M. de C., Travassos Jr., X. L. and Tilp, J. (2019). A universidade para a indústria do futuro, *Revista Eletrônica de Extensão*, **16**(33). Disponível em: https://periodicos.ufsc.br/index.php/ extensio/article/view/61861> (acesso em 26 ago. 2020).

21. Schwab, K. (2016). *A Quarta Revolução Industrial*. São Paulo: Edipro.

22. The Guardian (2020). Lockdowns around the world bring rise in domestic violence. Disponível em: https://www.theguardian.com/society/2020/mar/28/lockdowns-world-rise-domestic-violence?CMP=Share_iOSApp_Other> (acesso em 27 ago. 2020).

23. Yao, H., Chen, J.-H., Zhao, M., Qiu, J.-Y., Koenen, K. C., Stewart, Robert, S., Mellor, D. and Xu, Y.-F. (2020). Mitigating mental health consequences during the COVID-19 outbreak: lessons from China, *Psychiatry Clin. Neurosci.*, **74**(7), pp. 407–408. Disponível em: https://onlinelibrarywiley.ez101.periodicos.capes.gov.br/doi/full/10.1111/pcn.13018> (acesso em 27 ago. 2020).

24. Floridi, L. (2018). Soft ethics and the governance of the digital, *Philos. Technol.*, **31**, pp. 1–8.

25. Privacy versus public health (1 May 2020). UWIRE Text, p. 1. Gale Academic OneFile, https://link-gale.ez101.periodicos.capes.gov.br/apps/doc/A622481757/AONE?u=capes&sid=AONE&xid=72a4719e (accessed 24 June 2020).

26. Jamrozik, E. and Selgelid, M. J. (2020). COVID-19 – human challenge studies: ethical issues, *Lancet Infect. Dis.*, [Online]. https://doi.org/10.1016/ S1473-3099(20)30438-2.

27. Schwab, K. and Malleret, T. (2020). *COVID-19: The Great Reset.* Switzerland: Forum Publishing; World Economic Forum (Livro em formato Kindle).

28. Schwab, K. and Davis, N. (2018). *Aplicando a Quarta Revolução Industrial.* Tradução Daniel Moreira Miranda. São Paulo: Edipro.

Chapter 12

Physical Barrier against COVID-19: Materials to Inhibit or Eliminate the Virus

Alessandro Estarque de Oliveira, Karine Machry,
Bruno José Chiaramonte de Castro, Gustavo Cardoso da Mata,
André Bernardo, Vádila Giovana Guerra, and
Mônica Lopes Aguiar

Federal University of São Carlos Rodovia Washington Luís, km 235, 13565-905,
São Carlos, SP, Brazil
mlaguiar@ufscar.br

The severe acute respiratory syndrome caused by the new coronavirus (SARS-CoV-2) started in Wuhan, Hubei Province, China, in late 2019, and spread quickly across the world, being declared a pandemic by the World Health Organization (WHO) on March 11, 2020 [109]. SARS-CoV-2 viruses have a spherical shape in general and some pleomorphism, with diameters ranging from 60 nm to 140 nm and with spikes of 9 to 12 nm over their surface [115], and the aerosols produced by people when they breathe, talk, or cough may contain pieces of genetic material from the virus, which float easily in the air. As the pandemic progressed, a continuing shortage of evidence on the SARS-CoV-2 transmission routes resulted in several changes to the infection prevention and control guidelines.

Living with COVID-19: Economics, Ethics, and Environmental Issues
Edited by Chaudhery Mustansar Hussain and Gustavo Marques da Costa
Copyright © 2022 Jenny Stanford Publishing Pte. Ltd.
ISBN 978-981-4877-78-7 (Hardcover), 978-1-003-16828-7 (eBook)
www.jennystanford.com

One was released by the WHO on July 10, 2020, after an open letter from scientists specialized in the spread of diseases through the air requested updates on how the respiratory disease spreads, calling for the inclusion of the COVID-19 transmission over air [108]. However, more research is needed to confirm such evidence. Since the virus can be found suspended in air, the use of filter media as physical barriers capable of containing its spread is of vital importance. In this scenario, several tissues appeared to reduce the spread of the virus. Fabrics with the application of metal nanoparticles of silver, copper, and titanium, among others, stand out for inhibiting the spread of the virus since these nanoparticles are known for their biocidal and virucidal effects. Therefore, the dissemination can be controlled through the application of these filter media in internal ventilation systems, such as simple air conditioners. The supplied air must be clean in terms of particulate matter, gases, and pathogens (such as viruses, bacteria, and fungus spores), especially in hospitals and health-care facilities. This chapter presents an updated scenario about air quality standards worldwide and filter performance tests. SARS-CoV-2 is analyzed as a nanoparticle with regard to its dynamics in aerosols and its deposition in fibrous materials. The main mechanisms of deposition and collection of nanometric particles in fibers and the increase in the collection efficiency of these agents by nanofibers are presented. The main studies on bioaerosol filtration and current research about biocidal and virucidal materials are addressed.

12.1 Current Standards in Air Filtration

According to estimates from the World Health Organization (WHO), 90% of the global population breathes polluted air and about 7 million people die prematurely every year due to the combined effects of ambient and household air pollution [107]. Air pollutants can be classified as gaseous pollutants, such as ozone, nitrogen oxides, sulfur dioxide, and carbon monoxide, or particulate pollutants, if they are present in the atmosphere as suspended solid or liquid particles. Particulate pollutants have truly diverse sizes, from a few nanometers to some micrometers, and also very diverse chemical compositions, depending on their source [105].

Unless they are soluble in water, gaseous air pollutants deeply penetrate the human respiratory system. Exposure to ozone has been related to respiratory and cardiovascular diseases [72], susceptibility to respiratory infections is increased by nitrogen oxides [48], ventilatory capacity and shortness of breath are felt after the first minutes of exposure to sulfur dioxide [105], and carbon monoxide reduces the oxygen-carrying capacity of the blood and can lead to permanent damage to the central nervous system [106].

Particulate pollutants with diameters smaller than 10 μm (PM$_{10}$) can penetrate the human airways. The smaller their sizes, the greater the probability of their reaching the bronchiole and alveoli, affecting gas exchange and causing severe respiratory diseases. Particles with diameters smaller than 2.5 μm (PM$_{2.5}$) are especially dangerous and, once in the alveoli, there is a great chance that they will pass into the circulatory system. Then, they are transported via blood throughout the body, which may be related to the development of heart diseases, strokes, and cancers [16, 51, 57, 68, 90] and decrease in cognitive functions [2, 76, 96].

Pathogenic agents, such as viruses, bacteria, and fungus spores can also be considered particulate air pollutants, since they are easily suspended due to their tiny size: 20–400 nm for viruses, 0.2–2 μm for bacteria, and 2–8 μm for fungus spores [45, 95, 114]. To date, the main known way of transmission of the new coronavirus (SARS-CoV-2) is through droplets expelled from infected people when they cough, sneeze, or speak. These droplets may contain the virus and can be breathed in by unprotected close people or can settle in close surfaces like tables, handrails and other objects, from where they can contaminate other people later. However, the possibility of the virus to stay suspended in the air for longer periods of time and to travel further distances, especially in poorly ventilated closed rooms, is not discarded, mainly after recent reported outbreaks of COVID-19 in restaurants and offices [108], which brings the world's attention to air quality standards; heating, ventilation, and air-conditioning (HVAC) systems; and the types of fabrics used in such systems. Airborne diseases become an important issue, especially for crowded places like hospitals, public transport, markets, offices, and schools [8]. Therefore, protection against air contamination is required by improving the indoor infrastructure of buildings to protect patients, health-care workers, caregivers, and people in general.

On the basis of extensive scientific evidence and reports on air pollution and its health consequences, the WHO offers air quality guidelines that are consulted worldwide and support the authorities responsible for public policies related to air pollution in their countries [105]. The current guidelines for particulates and some of the most important gaseous pollutants are summarized in Table 12.1, along with the air quality standards currently adopted by the United States, the European Union, Brazil, China, South Africa, and Australia. The averaging time is the period over which the average value is determined.

The use of fabrics as physical barriers to filter the air with the objective of protecting human health is a millenary practice and the most commonly used method for HVAC systems. The barrier, known as a filter medium, must be permeable to air and efficiently retain the suspended particles [20, 78]. Careful selection of the filter medium to be used in HVAC systems is of extreme importance to guarantee high indoor air quality and consequently protect human health. In this context, defining common methods of characterizing filter media around the world is crucial, mainly for determining the collection efficiencies by particle size and the resistance to airflow, which is the loss of static pressure caused by the filter and filter loading.

The international standard UNE-EN ISO 16890:2016 defines an efficiency classification system of air filters for general ventilation on the basis of their particulate matter (PM) collection efficiency by particle size. Collection efficiencies of particles in the size ranges of 0.3–1 μm (ePM_1), 0.3–2.5 μm ($ePM_{2.5}$), and 0.3–10 μm (ePM_{10}) are used as the classification criteria. The standard also describes the bench-scale test rig, the required equipment and materials, and the procedures to measure the fractional collection efficiencies and convert them into the suggested reporting system. The airflow rate used in the tests are in the range of 0.25–1.5 m^3 s^{-1}, and the nominal face area is 0.61 m × 0.61 m. The collection efficiency of particles in the size range of 0.3–1 μm is assessed from a liquid-phase aerosol of diethyl-hexyl-sebacate, while a potassium chloride

Table 12.1 Current WHO air quality guidelines and maximum allowed concentrations of air pollutants in the US, EU, Brazil, China, South Africa, and Australia

Pollutant	Averaging time	WHO[a,b]	USA[c]	EU[d]	Brazil[e]	China[f]	South Africa[g]	Australia[h]
PM_{10} ($\mu g\,m^{-3}$)	Annual	20	–	40	40	70	40	–
	24 hours	50	150	50	120	150	75	50
$PM_{2.5}$ ($\mu g\,m^{-3}$)	Annual	10	15	25	20	35	–	8
	24 hours	25	35	–	60	75	–	25
Total suspended particles ($\mu g\,m^{-3}$)	Annual	–	–	–	80	200	–	–
Ozone ($\mu g\,m^{-3}$)	24 hours	–	–	–	240	300	–	–
	8 hours	100	138	120	140	160	120	–
	4 hours	–	–	–	–	–	–	157
	1 hour	–	–	–	–	200	–	197
NO_2 ($\mu g\,m^{-3}$)	Annual	40	100	40	60	40	40	57
	24 hours	–	–	–	–	80	–	–
	1 hour	200	189	200	260	200	200	226
SO_2 ($\mu g\,m^{-3}$)	Annual	–	–	–	40	60	50	52
	24 hours	20	–	125	125	150	125	209
	3 hours	–	1309	–	–	–	–	–
	1 hour	–	196	350	–	500	350	524
	10 min.	500	–	–	–	–	500	–

(*Contd.*)

Table 12.1 *(Contd.)*

Pollutant	Averaging time	WHO[a,b]	USA[c]	EU[d]	Brazil[e]	China[f]	South Africa[g]	Australia[h]
CO (mg m^{-3})	24 hours	7	–	–	–	4	–	–
	8 hours	10	10	10	10	–	10	10
	1 hour	35	40	–	–	10	30	–
	15 min.	100	–	–	–	–	–	–
Pb (µg m^{-3})	Annual	–	–	0.5	0.5	0.5	0.5	0.5
	3 months	–	0.15	–	–	–	–	–

[a]World Health Organization (WHO) (2006). Air quality guidelines: global update 2005. World Health Organization, Denmark.

[b]World Health Organization (WHO) (2010). WHO guidelines for indoor air quality: selected pollutants. World Health Organization, Denmark.

[c]United Stated Environmental Protection Agency. NAAQS table. Available at: <https://www.epa.gov/criteria-air-pollutants/naaqs-table> [accessed on July 29, 2020).

[d]European Commission. Environment. Air quality standards. Available at: <https://ec.europa.eu/environment/air/ quality/standards.htm > (accessed on July 29, 2020).

[e]Ministry of the Environment. National Environment Council. Resolution no. 491, November 19, 2018. Available at: <http://www2.mma. gov.br/port/conama/legiabre.cfm?codlegi=740> (accessed on July 29, 2020).

[f]Ministry of Ecology and Environment of the People's Republic of China. Ambient air quality standards (GB3095-2012). Available at: <http://english.mee.gov.cn/Resources/standards/Air_Environment/quality_standard1/201605/W020160511506615956495.pdf>[accessed on July 29, 2020].

[g]Department of Environmental Affairs. National environmental management: air quality act, 2004 (Act No. 39 of 2004). National ambient air quality standards. Available at: <https://www.gov.za/sites/default/files/gcis_document/201409/328161210.pdf>[accessed on July 29, 2020).

[h]Department of Agriculture, Water and the Environment. National standards for criteria air pollutants 1 in Australia. Available at: <https://www.environment.gov.au/protection/publications/factsheet-national-standards-criteria-air-pollutants-australia>[accessed on July 29, 2020).

(KCl) solution is used to evaluate the collection efficiency of particles in the size range of 1–10 μm. An optical particle spectrometer is used to count particles upstream and downstream the filter medium and thus provide the data required to calculate the fractional collection efficiencies.

A test method for evaluating the air permeability of fabrics that can be applied in air filtration devices is described by the standard ASTM D737-18 [5]. The standard circular test area is 38.30 cm^2, but alternate areas, such as 5, 6.45, and 100 cm^2, can also be used. The perpendicular airflow rate must be steady and provide pressure differentials of 100–2500 Pa between the two faces of the textile being tested. A flowmeter and a manometer are used to measure the airflow rate at the pressure differential specified in the material description, or at 125 Pa, if such information is not available. In SI units, values of air permeability are recorded as cm^3 s^{-1} cm^{-2}.

The performance of air cleaning devices in their end use installed configuration can be evaluated following the procedure described in the standard UNE-EN ISO 29462:2013. The collection efficiencies by particle size and the resistance to airflow are assessed by field testing of the device. Particles in the size range of 0.3–5 μm are counted by an optical counter, while the resistance to airflow is measured using a manometer.

Optical particle spectrometers, such as those described in UNE-EN ISO 16890:2016 and UNE-EN ISO 29462:2013 to assess the collection efficiency of airborne particles, are not suitable when the particles of interest have diameters smaller than 300 nm, which would probably be the case if the filter medium collection performance was being evaluated for viruses, like the SARS-CoV-2. The most commonly employed technique for measuring the concentration of particles in the size range of 3–1000 nm is based on electrical mobility analysis, using a device called scanning mobility particle sizer (SMPS). The electrical mobility distribution of the particles is measured and further converted into the number size distribution, since electrical mobility is a function of particle size and charge [15]. The use of an SMPS to determine the number concentration and size distribution of nanosized aerosols is described by UNE-EN ISO 28439:2011.

12.2 Physical Barriers in Filter Media

Particles are removed from a gas with the help of collection devices. The suitability of such devices is determined on the basis of their efficiency for a specific size range, besides cost-benefit requirements, energy consumption, and specificities of the process, such as high temperatures or severe humidity conditions: cyclonic separators operate with high efficiency only for particles greater than 10 μm, Venturi scrubbers efficiently remove particles above 5 μm, and electrostatic precipitators efficiently collect particles greater than 0.01 μm. High-efficiency particulate arrestance (HEPA) filters are generally used to capture particles smaller than 0.1 μm, while membrane filters are used for particles smaller than 20 μm; paper and cloth filter media efficiently collect particles with diameters greater than 5 μm, and industrial bag filters efficiently collect particles greater than 0.05 μm [97].

Different deposition mechanisms are involved in the removal of particles from air (Fig. 12.1), and their efficiency depends strongly on the particle properties, such as size, mass, and electrical permittivity. The main deposition mechanisms are interception, inertial impaction, diffusion, electrostatic attraction, and gravity [36]. In interception, particles are thought as spheres with size but not mass. Hence, they flow with the gas streamlines toward the collection body (the fibers in the case of collection by filter media); the particle traveling in a streamline close enough to the fiber surface can be captured by it if the distance between the particle and the fiber is less than the particle radius. In inertial impaction, particles with a considerable mass, when traveling along with the gas streamline that flows toward the fiber, can be collected by the fiber surface if their inertia prevents them from deviating from the fiber. Particles with a considerable mass can also be collected by gravity depending on their terminal velocity and the main gas velocity. There can be electrostatic attraction, or even repulsion, between the fiber and the particles and even between particles, depending on the electrical charges carried or induced between these bodies. Finally, particles can be captured by diffusion when their size is close to the mean free path of the gas and they

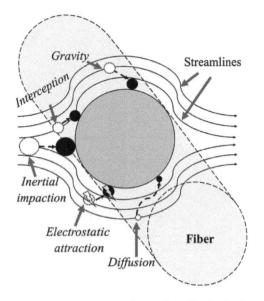

Figure 12.1 Representation of particles before (dashed spheres) and after (full black spheres) the influence of the collection mechanisms involving a single fiber (light-gray cylinder with dark-gray cross section).

collide with the gas molecules, exhibiting random movement due to Brownian motion; in this case, an interception mechanism due exclusively to diffusion and not related to the streamlines of the gas must be considered [26, 36, 94].

The collection efficiency of a filter medium is determined by the efficiency of these deposition mechanisms, involving the efficiency of each fiber, besides the adhesion between particles and fibers and cohesion between the particles. Other variables lead the performance of the process, such as gas velocity, environmental conditions (pressure, temperature, and humidity of the gas stream), and even structural properties of the filter media, such as thickness, filtering area, and porosity, the last one not only related to the collection of the particles but also responsible for resistance to the gas flow and hence for the power consumption of the process [36].

To show an overview of how the deposition mechanisms act on a wide range of particle sizes, Fig. 12.2 shows the dimensionless form (0 to 1) of the efficiencies of the deposition mechanisms and

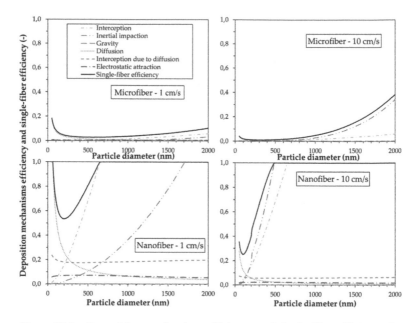

Figure 12.2 Deposition mechanism efficiency and single-fiber efficiency for a microfiber and a nanofiber at 1 and 10 cm/s.

the single-fiber efficiency for the collection of NaCl particles from 50 nm to 2 µm (or 2000 nm) in air (25°C and 101,325 Pa) at different face velocities, for a micrometric-size fiber (10 µm) and a nanometric-size fiber (500 nm). The properties of the particles and the air were obtained from Refs. [25, 84, 85], and the efficiency models were obtained from Hinds [36] using an extended form of the Kuwabara model [113] and the correlation of Flagan and Seinfeld [30] for the Cunningham factor. An electrically neutralized aerosol was considered. So the derivation of Wiedensohler [104] from the Fuchs model was used to obtain a Boltzmann distribution of electrical charges. The porosity was fixed at a high value (0.9) for both fibers for didactical purposes.

The efficiencies of the deposition mechanisms were irrisory for the particle size range evaluated for the microfiber at 1 cm s^{-1} of air, except for the diffusion mechanism, which presented an efficiency of 0.18 (or 18%) for 50 nm particles and whose efficiency decreased with the particle size up to $\sim$1 μm, providing an efficiency of 0.1 (or 10%) for a 2 μm particle. The interception and the impaction increased with the particle diameter, being, respectively, 6 and 3% for a 2 μm particle. The single-fiber efficiency was composed mostly of the diffusion mechanism of particles of up to 500 nm diameter. The increase of the velocity from 1 to 10 cm s^{-1} enhanced the impaction and decreased the diffusion, being, respectively, 34 and 0% for a 2 μm particle.

However, the interactions between the particles and the fibers began involving other mechanisms for the case of the nanofibers, especially the interception due to the diffusional mechanism (blue lines) for particles up to 600 nm and whose prominence increased with the reduction of the fiber size. Nanoparticle behavior lies between the transition-to-continuum and the free-molecule flow regime, while both particles and nanofibers have sizes close to the mean free path of the gas, favoring Brownian motion and subsequently diffusion and diffusion-promoted interception [36, 52, 113]. At the lowest air velocity, single-fiber efficiency was equal to the maximum for 600 nm particles, while there was a minimum single-fiber efficiency for particles of $\sim$200 nm with air at 1 cm s^{-1} (53.4%) due to the superposition of the mechanisms, while the increase of the velocity displaced this minimum to particles 90 nm in diameter (25.4%). In relation to electrostatic attraction and interception due to diffusion, both remained almost the same for particles of 200 nm diameter, being respectively equal to 7 and 18% for air at 1 cm $^{-1}$ and respectively equal to 2 and 6% for air at 10 cm s^{-1}. Efficiency by gravity was irrisory for all the cases.

These results attested to the importance of using filter media made of nanofibers to collect ultrafine particles, either in face masks and protective clothing or for air purifiers. Nanofibers have been produced generally by electrospinning of polymeric solutions or melts and have been applied in protective clothing and face masks. These have high breathability and give protection against chemical and biological attack [31, 82, 100], as well as in the filtration of ultrafine and nanometric particles from air streams [22, 61, 62], in which there may be biocidal agents impregnated in the fibers [12, 13, 63], as will be explored further.

12.3 Filtration of Bioaerosols

Viruses, bacteria, fungi and their spores and toxins, pollen, and fragments of insects and vestiges of animal and plant cells are categorized as bioaerosols, and their collection demands more attention and restrictions due to their ability to reproduce and to exert metabolic activity even after their capture. In addition, the small mass and inertia of the viral particulate hinder its sampling and collection with methods dependent on inertial and gravitational mechanisms [33], as explored in the discussion of the efficiencies presented in Fig. 12.2 for nanoparticles. Thus, filtration is presented as a process of gas-solid separation that is more efficient and viable in the mitigation of the spread of pathogenic agents, either by using face masks—specially to retain contaminated fluid from the user— or by using air conditioners and HVAC systems [98]. Since Chapter 4 is already focused on face masks to retain bioaerosols, the following content explores the application of filtration phenomena in these latter devices.

SARS-CoV-2 viruses have a spherical shape in general and some pleomorphism, with diameters ranging from 60 nm to 140 nm and spikes 9–12 nm in size over their surface [89, 115]. They can be dispersed in the atmosphere by micrometric droplets expelled by the human body during coughing and sneezing. However, saliva droplets dispersed in the air can dehydrate and shrink according to the nonvolatile materials present in their constitution, such as enzymes, sugars, DNA, and electrolytes, in such a way that 12–21 µm droplets can dehydrate into 4 µm droplets, depending on the environmental conditions and the source of expulsion [93]. On the other hand, there is the possibility of the virus coalescing into particles greater than $PM_{2.5}$ when they are dispersed in the atmosphere [91]. Rohit et al. [86] evaluated the setting velocity of droplets of 0.1 to 100 µm and associated variations of this property to environmental humidity, which could cause changes in the evaporation rate of the water and lead to the dehydration of the droplets in the air. The authors then pointed out that the particulate containing pathogenic agents (like SARS-CoV-2) could remain in air for longer times in locations of the globe with low temperatures and humidity. The use of face masks was emphasized as an essential action to mitigate the transmission of viruses in these areas, besides hand hygiene and social distancing. In fact, this action is recommended especially in closed environments without mechanical ventilation, as reported by the work of Zhang et al. [112], which modeled the dispersion of SARS-CoV-2 in the seafood market of Wuhan (China), from where the virus has allegedly spread. On the basis of these results, researchers stated that social distancing of 1–2 m may not be enough to restrain the spread of the virus and that the success in reducing the transmission of pathogenic agents is associated directly to the retention of $PM_{2.5}$ and PM_{10} [7, 11, 91].

The presence of air-conditioning systems decreases the concentration of airborne bioaerosols over time in closed rooms and vehicles, as reported by Jo and Lee [44]. The authors verified a decrease in the bioaerosol concentration over 5–15 min. after the air conditioning was turned on in a seminar room prior to use. They also verified the differences in the bioaerosol concentration in the air inside different cars located in an outdoor environment after their engines were started, achieving a maximum bacterial concentration (2550 CFU m^{-3}) 46-fold higher in the outdoor environment than that measured inside the vehicle background concentration (55 CFU m^{-3}). In the meantime, Brochot et al. [14] tested the nanoparticle collection performances (efficiency and pressure drop) of using several commercial filters applied in air conditioners in order to evaluate the most penetrating particle size (MPPS) range. The researchers attested that the size range from 150 to 500 nm better estimated the performance of filters collecting nanoparticles than the one provided by the ANSI/ASHRAE 52.2 standard [6], equal to 300 nm.

While there are several works on manufacturing nanofiber filter media for air filtration applications in general [38, 61, 65], some studies have focused on the production of nanofibers for air-conditioning systems. In these cases, it is possible to apply additives in the production of these filter media or even the impregnation of these materials in commercial filters, in order to enhance the deposition mechanisms for nanoparticles achieved with the nanofibers, as explained earlier, with biocidal effects provided by these additives, which will be further explored. Rosa et al. [87]

impregnated silver nanoparticles (Ag NPs) in commercial fabric filters used in air conditioners in order to provide biocidal effects and to reduce the bioaerosol concentration in indoor environments. The enhanced filter media was able to inhibit the growth of microorganisms encountered in a bathroom and that were retained by the fibers by up to 70%.

HVAC systems are special setups for air conditioning, and they are related to the concept of clean rooms, which are indoor environments with different categorizations and whose particle concentration in the internal air is strictly controlled for each range of particle size, as regulated by ISO 146441-1. According to this standard, an ISO Class 1 room must control the concentration of 0.1 and 0.2 μm particles in the indoor environment up to the maximum of 10 and 2 particles/m^3, respectively (for more details on indoor air quality, please refer to Tan [98]). In these HVAC systems, particles can be collected by a combination of filter media and electrostatic precipitators to guarantee the highest efficiency [74, 50], but HEPA filters may be preferable instead of electrostatic precipitators since electrostatic precipitators, as much as air ionizers, may produce ozone and subsequently volatile organic compounds, like terpenes and aldehydes [101].

Mechanical ventilation and air conditioning of indoor environments must be efficient. Otherwise, they could help to spread the virus through mechanically created airflow currents [64]. In addition, care must be taken about the cleanliness and expiration of air filters in air-conditioning units, whether in buildings or cars, in order to avoid contamination by pathogenic agents, which can grow on the surface of the fibers after the particle collection depending on the environmental circumstances; hence disinfection or exchange is mandatory [32, 49, 60].

12.4 Filter Media in Removing Airborne Virus

As mentioned previously, the removal of airborne viruses is challenging due to their small size. In this context, Konda and coworkers [53] tested various common fabrics as filter media against the coronavirus, such as cotton, silk, chiffon, and flannel.

Natural fibers retain less static charge than polyester woven fabrics due to their higher water adsorption properties [75].

In filtration, nonwoven fabrics present advantages when compared to woven fabrics, such as no yarn slippage, increase of air permeability, higher bacterial filtration efficiency, and low manufacture cost [54]. Chellamani and collaborators [19] suggested that nonwoven filter media can be more effective in filtration than common fabrics, since they normally exhibit better barrier properties due the interactions between the PM and the fibers of the filter media [19].

Recently, filters composed of nanofibers have been produced by electrospinning and they have been applied to air purification with high efficiency [3]. The electrospinning technique is cost effective and a simple way to create fibrous membranes, it being possible to vary properties of the fibers as per their porosities and diameters [79]. Electrospun nanofibers are highly suitable for filtration applications due to their high specific area and good pore interconnectivity, with well-defined small pores [92]. High specific areas also improve the collection mechanism for small particles, like the SARS-CoV-2. Diffusion is the main filtration phenomenon for the severe acute respiratory syndrome (SARS) family due to their small diameters [66]. Mechanical capture by interception is also relevant [58] for particles of this size, as mentioned in Sections 12.2 and 12.3.

The electrospinning technique consists in creating electrostatic polymer fibers from polymer solutions or melts using a high voltage applied between a capillary tube or needle and a collector with controlled deposition on the target [1]. In the case of polymer solutions, the solvent evaporates and nano- or microsize fibers reach the collector. The filtration theory dictates that a reduction in fiber size leads to improvement in filtration efficiency [55] due to the increase of surface area. Various parameters can be modified to control the nanofiber size, such as the polymer solution properties and environmental and process conditions. Variables such as viscosity, surface tension, conductivity, room temperature, and humidity also affect the morphology and formation of the fibers. Process parameters like voltage, space nozzle, and collector geometry also have a pivotal influence on the filtration performance [3].

Leung and Sun [59] varied the fiber diameter of polyvinylidene fluoride (PVDF) nanofibers (fibers of average diameters 84 nm, 191 nm, 349 nm, and 525 nm) and compared their collection efficiency. They performed tests with sodium chloride aerosols 50–500 nm in size to simulate COVID-19 and possible combined aerosols and observed that the reduction of the fiber size led to an increase in the collection efficiency. The authors produced fibers with average diameters of 525 nm, 349 nm, 191 nm, and 84 nm, which had collection efficiencies of 39.6%, 45.3%, 51.8%, and 61.9%, respectively. The MPPS was 280 nm for fibers of 525 nm and 200 nm for fibers of 84 nm.

Almeida et al. [4] also used NaCl crystals to simulate airborne coronavirus, with particle size ranging from 7 nm to 299 nm and obtained efficiencies of almost 100%. They used fibers of cellulose acetate (CA), which is a biodegradable material, with cationic surfactant cetylpyridinium bromide (CPB). The goal was to produce nontoxic and biodegradable fibers instead of using common polymers. The addition of surfactants to CA aimed to improve mechanical and thermal resistance of the material without the material losing its biodegradable capability. The CA/CBP electrospun fiber filter was also challenged with environment aerosol and provided higher collection efficiency for $PM_{2.5}$ than commercial quartz fiber-based filters. The fiber, with a diameter of 375 nm, also retained carbonaceous particles from biomass combustion with an efficiency of 90% for $PM_{2.5}$.

Das et al. [24] focused on biodegradable materials to avoid the production of more environmental pollutants and produced membranes with electrospun nanofiber from gluten biopolymer. The material was carbonized at over 700°C in order to generate the network structure of the filter medium. The natural compound lanasol was added to the nanofibers to make the gluten plastics microbe resistant.

Independently of the production technique of the nanofibers, they are not evenly distributed on the substrate [9]. The thinner part of the substrate can create a preferential pathway to airflow due to the lower resistance, which would reduce collection efficiency. One way to avoid the effects of nonuniformity of the substrate is using multiple layers of nanofiber [77].

However, the increase in the filtration efficiency can bring together an increase in pressure drop, increasing filtration costs. One approach to reduce this variable is to improve the distribution of nanofibers in multilayers, which would increase efficiency without increasing the pressure drop too much. Each thin nanofiber layer can be attached to a permeable substrate (a module) with a large number of macropores dispersed in the layers of the filter medium [58].

Yu et al. [110] considered the fact that the airborne SARS-CoV-2 cannot survive at temperatures above 70°C and produced filters based on heated nickel (Ni) foams, aiming to catch and inactivate the virus. The authors verified that up to 99.8% of the aerosolized coronavirus was caught and eliminated in one pass across the filter, heated up to 200°C. Efficiency of the Ni-foam-based filter to catch and kill 99.9% airborne spores of *Bacillus anthracis* was also tested. They folded the Ni-foam-based filter to improve its mechanical resistance and to create a hot zone between the curves of the folded foam, as shown in Fig. 12.3. The authors varied the thickness of the filter by folding it, from 1.6 mm (flat form) to 1.6 cm (folded form), increasing the surface area of the filter media. Airborne filtration by a filter media with a high surface area can be positive due to the increase of interactions between the foam and the particles, but can lead to an enhancement of the filtration costs. According to the experimental procedure, the airflow was forced through the filter and the air remained in the hot zone for enough time for the

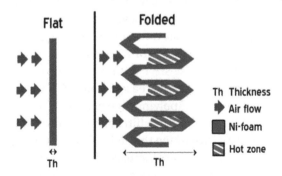

Figure 12.3 Schematic side view of the flat Ni foam and folded Ni foam.

coronavirus to be inactivated but not long enough for the air to be heated.

A work worthy of mention is that of Park et al. [74]. The authors presented a new method to test the antiviral efficiency of air filters against airborne infectious viruses. Tests were performed, and the authors concluded that this methodology can be efficiently used to test antiviral effect in filter media without the need of aerosolizing the virus. This methodology can minimize procedure risks and exposure to pathogens (SARS-CoV-2, H1N1, etc.) for the manipulators. The authors compared their method with air media test, using the noninfectious viruses' bacteriophages MS2, T1, and T4 and, as an infectious virus, H1N1. An inquiry was made to ensure that the relationship does not depend on the virus species. It was successfully tested with various antiviral filters, obtaining their capabilities under continuous airflow condition.

12.5 Electrostatically-Assisted Air Filtration

The presence of electrostatic charges in the fibers usually improves particle removal efficiency without increasing the pressure drop and, in some cases, it even decreases the pressure drop. Charged particles are attracted by fibers with an opposite charge, while neutral particles form a dipole, induced by the charges of the fibers [56]. Kravtsov et al. [56] worked with melt-spun polypropylene fibers treated by a corona discharge. They observed that the charge is trapped in the material, which makes the polypropylene fibers hold the induced electret state for several months.

Hyun et al. [39] studied the effect of the corona discharge in MS2 bacteriophages with a mean size of 27.6 nm, much smaller than the coronavirus of the smallest size. With a gas ionizer, the filtration efficiency of bacteriophages increased from 56.5% to 63.5% at a flow velocity of 0.3 m s^{-1}. Applying an external electric field of 2 kV cm^{-1}, an increment of 71.7% on filtration efficiency was obtained. At low velocities (e.g., breathing through a face mask), the collection efficiency of electrostatic filters increases [23]. The higher residence time allows more interactions between the aerosol particles and the filter fibers. For particles above 15 nm, the increments in efficiency due to the presence of air ions and electric field were evident. However, significant changes in the collection efficiency of particles below 15 nm were not observed since small particles acquire lower charge numbers and are difficult to measure.

Leung and Sun [58, 59] also evaluated multilayer charged structures to retain the coronavirus. Using NaCl crystals to simulate the bioaerosol of SARS-CoV-2, they tested a charged multilayer filter, produced by electrospun PVDF, and compared it with an uncharged multilayer filter. The collection efficiency of the MPPS increased from 24% for the uncharged filter to 48% for the charged filter, with the shift of the MPPS from 150 nm to 70 nm, respectively. For small aerosols, diffusion is stronger in nanofibers than in microfibers, where the diffusion is much subdued. To capture nanoaerosols, as discussed in Section 12.2, microfiber filters depend primarily on the electrostatic effect because of the weak diffusion phenomenon. Charged nanofiber filters present the advantage of capturing aerosols by both effects. In this context, pathogen microorganisms like viruses can be captured by the fibers and tend to remain infectious for hours or up to several days. To diminish the possibility of contamination, Section 12.6 will talk about how to reduce these pathogens from fibers.

12.6 Biocidal and Virucidal Agents to Control the Spread of Diseases Applied to Air Filtration

During the pandemic of COVID-19, the world started a race against time for materials that could inhibit or eliminate the SARS-CoV-2 and also other types of enveloped and nonenveloped viruses from surfaces. As already mentioned, the spread of SARS-CoV-2 virus occurs by the emission of droplets. The smallest droplets (<5 μm) can move quite a distance and remain airborne longer, while the largest ones (greater than 5 μm) fall rapidly to the ground after being produced [67] and remain infectious on surfaces. Besides the SARS-CoV-2, there are other types of pathogen microorganisms that can be in by air, including fungi, bacteria, and other viruses. Transmission of airborne infections occurs by droplet nuclei; it refers to the particle of an evaporated wet droplet, with diameters less than 5 μm, that remains infectious carries pathogens such as varicella-zoster virus, rubella, tuberculosis, measles virus, influenza (the flu), Middle East respiratory syndrome, and SARS.

At the end of July 2020, there were 16 million cases of SARS-CoV-2 and more than 650,000 deaths according to the Situation Report – 190 of the WHO [109]. The spread of the virus was very fast; it began on December 31, 2019 in Wuhan, China. The rapid spread of the virus encouraged several researchers to explore the contamination process once several services were suspended, such as international flights, to contain the virus. A study was developed in a small-scale using CFD, aiming to understand the spread of SARS in an airline cabin. It was shown that the highest concentration of contamination was along two rows from the infected passenger but the contamination can reach a passenger sitting seven rows from the infected individual by the movement body along the aisle [67]. In this context, especially in longer flights, one contaminated passenger is capable of contaminating many others even far from him or her and the spread is intensified with the movement of people in the aisle, such as stewards. The spread of the virus can be diminished, but not eliminated, with the use of equipment such as masks. SARS-CoV-2 has an average diameter of 100 nm, and masks such as the N95 respirator, which has 95% efficiency for particles between 100 nm and 300 nm [81], can be used. To contain the disease, a good alternative is the development of materials with biocidal and virucidal proprieties to be used in hospitals, by health-care workers, in masks, or even in filtration systems.

Nanoparticles (normally materials ranging from 1 nm to 100 nm) could be useful to prevent, eliminate, or even diminish the presence of pathogen microorganisms and to help prevent virus spread due to their modified optical, electronic, and mechanical proprieties when compared with the same material in bulk form [38]. The advantage of nanoparticles is their small size, which allows the use of a lower amount of mass than the bulk form, with a greater contact surface area (Fig. 12.4), bringing economic benefits. Several metals are used as nanoparticles in different areas. In this context, several areas have attracted the application of nanoparticles and most studies concerning COVID-19 involve the versatility, efficiency, and price

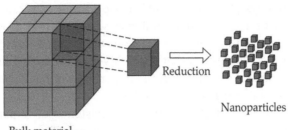

Bulk material

Figure 12.4 Increase in surface area due to the reduction in size from the bulk material to nanoparticles.

performance of these applications. Ag NPs have biocidal, fungicidal, and virucidal proprieties and they were widely employed in several applications, mostly to modify fabrics used personal protective equipment.

Tremiliosi and collaborators [99] developed a fabric modified with Ag NPs and tested the antiviral activity of the textile following the ISO 18184 determination. The authors found that the presence of Ag NPs led to a reduction by 99.99% of SARS-CoV-2 within 2–5 min. of coming in contact with the fabric. The same authors found 99.99% of inhibition to *Staphylococcus aureus*, *Escherichia coli*, and *Candida albicans*, indicating that Ag NPs are effective against virus, bacteria, and fungi. A company from Brazil has developed a product with Ag NPs that can eliminate 99.999% of enveloped and nonenveloped viruses [88]. The product can be used in the wiring and the dyeing process of several types of fabrics and can retain its efficiency for up to 70 washes. The company was sought to provide products for the fabrication of filter media, face masks, medical aprons, cleaning cloths, and inks and for several polymers, including toothbrushes and sponges [88]. This alternative can be useful for new products but not for existing ones.

In this context, a spray with Ag NPs was developed to be used as a disinfectant [17]. Lower concentrations of the nanoparticles led to a low cost, and the application of the spray can be easier, cheaper, and more effective than an alcohol gel. Also, the spray can be used in several applications, as cleaning facial protectors and contaminated surfaces, where coronavirus can remain infectious for several days [102] and at different pH levels at room ambient [21]. In plastic, stainless steel, and masks (inner layer), SARS-CoV-2 could be detected in low concentrations even after 4 days [21] and Neeltje et al. [71] showed that SARS-CoV-2 can remain active for 3 hours in aerosols, reminding of the importance of the development of materials with virucidal proprieties.

Warnes et al. [102] studied the persistence of a pathogenic human coronavirus 229E on common surfaces. The authors found that the inactivation of HuCoV-229E was directly proportional to the percentage of copper, indicating that this metal can also help in the war against the virus, especially the enveloped one. The same study showed that this pathogenic virus can remain infectious for at least 5 days in common surface materials, such as polytetrafluorethylene (Teflon), polyvinyl chloride, ceramic tiles, glass, silicone rubber, and stainless steel, while in copper alloy surfaces, this time was reduced to a few minutes [102]. Future studies aim to employ copper nanoparticles in inks and fabrics and even in alcohol gel to confer on them antimicrobial proprieties [43]. Up to the present moment, there has been no study with copper nanoparticles and SARS-CoV-2. What is known up to now is that copper nanoparticles interact with other species of coronaviruses and have bactericidal, fungicidal, and virucidal effect [10].

Many fabrics modified with nanoparticles have been created during the pandemic, but despite the fact that the use of nanoparticles covers several areas, scientists have also developed other methods to contain the spread of the disease. A revolutionary and curious study was the development of a cellular nanosponge to inhibit the infectivity of SARS-CoV-2 [111]. These nanosponges are developed with the cell membranes of the lung epithelial cells from humans and synthesized with poly(DL-lactic-*co*-glycolic acid). They were tested in vivo, and results showed that the nanosponges can be used in the lungs to neutralize the virus because they have the capability of attracting the viruses due to the receptors present in the structure that are the same receptors that the viruses depend on for cellular entry [111]. The idea of nanosponges is that they can be used to link the receptors of the virus before it reaches the lungs, thereby inhibiting the attack of SARS-CoV-2, or even other viruses, on lung cells. Due to the high surface area of nanoparticles, nanofibers, and nanosponges, this scale can be useful in several areas.

In the current COVID-19 pandemic, the modification of fabrics, masks, and even disinfectants with Ag NPs in the combat of SARS-CoV-2 was explored [17, 88, 99]. The use of biocidal and virucidal materials on surfaces is an alternative for reducing the transmission of infectious pathogenic diseases from a surface to an individual. However, you should be asking yourself, how does the transmission occur between the pathogenic microorganism and the nanoparticle or even a biocidal/virucidal surface?

The toxic effect that leads the pathogen microorganism to death is complex and can change with the material, shape, and size of the nanoparticle. Tremiliosi et al. [99] proposed that the mechanism between the bacteria (gram-positive and gram-negative) consists in the penetration of the Ag NPs into the cell membrane of these microorganisms and the Ag NPs' reaction with phosphorous and sulfur compounds due the release of Ag^+ ions from the nanoparticles to the cell membrane. Also, the presence of metal nanoparticles like Ag NPs can generate reactive oxygen species, leading to oxidative stress and cell damage. In viruses, the authors proposed that the first mechanism consists in binding of Ag NPs with the surface of the viruses. The second mechanism consists in the passage of the Ag NPs through the cell membrane and blockage of the transcription factor.

For the case of the human coronavirus HuCoV-229E and a surface of copper, the surfaces induce the liberation of copper ions, which results in the fragmentation of the viral genome, leading to irreversible inactivation of the virus [102]. The authors proposed a possible reaction between bacteria and copper surfaces, involving the copper ion and the bacteria generating oxygen radicals and multiple chain reactions, leading the bacteria to a "metabolic suicide." A study using epifluorescence microscopy to verify bacterial damage contested that copper ions interrupted the respiratory pathway and/or damaged the genomic DNA of the cell. This study concluded that the presence of copper ions on a surface does not affect the integrity of the cell membrane and, possibly, copper toxicity occurs in the same way in gram-negative bacteria, leading to the loss of genomic DNA and interruption of the respiration pathway of the bacteria [103].

Despite the toxic effect between nanoparticles and bacteria/viruses not being totally clear, several tests have shown that the presence of these particles reduces the growth of bacteria and inactivates viruses. In this context, the use of nanoparticles in filter media or fabrics or as disinfectants is an alternative to reduce the presence of pathogen microorganisms on surfaces.

12.7 Final Considerations

It is important to remember that currently the spread of COVID-19 is a big problem that the world is facing, and apart from SARS-CoV-2, there are other bacterial or viral agents that can be transmitted by aerosol droplets (<5 μm), such as *Mycobacterium tuberculosis*, a pathogenic bacterium of tuberculosis that usually attacks the lungs; the common flu, caused by influenza virus; varicella (chickenpox), caused by varicella-zoster virus; rubella, by rubella virus; and also coronaviruses, causing several respiratory syndrome, such as SARS, MERS, and COVID-19. The reduction of pathogens on surfaces is one way to fight against invisible microorganisms like viruses, bacteria, and fungi.

As shown in this chapter, there are several physical and biochemical mechanisms in air filtration that are important in order to optimize the retention of microorganisms like viruses, with diameters of approximately 100 nm. The adaptation of those fabrics employing nanoparticles is a good alternative to avoid the spread of SARS-CoV-2 and other pathogenic microorganisms, contributing to the fight against COVID-19 and possible future endemics and pandemics.

References

1. Ahn, Y. C., Park, S. K., Kim, G. T., Hwang Y. J., Lee, C. G., Shin, H. S. and Lee, J. K. (2006). Development of high efficiency nanofilters made of nanofibers, *Curr. Appl. Phys.*, **6**(6), pp. 1030–1035.

2. Ailshire, J., Karraker, A. and Clarke, P. (2017). Neighborhood social stressors, fine particulate matter air pollution, and cognitive function among older U.S. adults, *Soc. Sci. Med.*, **172**, pp. 56–63.

3. Aliabadi, M. (2017). Effect of electrospinning parameters on the air filtration performance using electrospun polyamide-6 nanofibers, *CICEQ*, **23**(4), pp. 441–446.

4. Almeida, D. S., Martins, L. D., Muniz, E. C., Rudke, A. P., Squizzato, R., Beal, A., Souza, P. R., Bonfim, D. P. F., Aguiar, M. L. and Gimenes, M. L. (2020). Biodegradable CA/CPB electrospun nanofibers for efficient retention of airborne nanoparticles, *Process Saf. Environ.*, **144**, pp. 177–185.

5. American Society for Testing and Materials (2018). *ASTM D737 – 18: Standard Test Method for Air Permeability of Textile Fabrics*. ASTM International: United States.

6. American Society of Heating, Refrigerating and Air-Conditioning Engineers (2017). *ANSI/ASHRAE Standard 52.2. Method of Testing General Ventilation Air-Cleaning Devices for Removal Efficiency by Particle Size*. ASHRAE: United States.

7. Amoatey, P., Omidvarborna, H., Baawain, M. S. and Al-Mamun, A. (2020). Impact of building ventilation systems and habitual indoor incense burning on SARS-CoV-2 virus transmissions in Middle Eastern countries, *Sci. Total Environ.*, **733**, p. 139356.

8. Balagna, C., Perero, S., Percivalle, E., Nepita, E. V. and Ferraris, M. (2020). Virucidal effect against coronavirus SARS-CoV-2 of a silver nanocluster/silica composite sputtered coating, *Open Ceram.*, **1**, p. 100006.

9. Barhate, R. S. and Ramakrishna, S. (2007). Nanofibrous filtering media: Filtration problems and solutions from tiny materials, *J. Membr. Sci.*, **296**, pp. 1–8.

10. Bogdanovi, U., Lazi, V., Vodnik, V., Budimir, M., Markovi, Z. and Dimitrijevi, S. (2014). Copper nanoparticles with high antimicrobial activity, *Mater. Lett.*, **128**, pp. 75–78.

11. Borak, J. (2020). Airborne transmission of COVID-19, *Occup. Med.*, **70**(5), pp. 297–299.

12. Bortolassi, A. C. C., Guerra, V. G., Aguiar, M. L., Soussan, L., Cornu, D., Miele, P. and Bechelany, M. (2019). Composites based on nanoparticle and panelectrospun nanofiber membranes for air filtrationand bacterial removal, *Nanomaterials*, **9**, p. 1740.

13. Bortolassi, A. C. C., Nagarajan, S., Lima, B. A., Guerra, V. G., Aguiar, M. L., Huon, V., Soussan, L., Cornu, D., Miele, P. and Bechelany, M. (2019). Efficient nanoparticles removal and bactericidal action of electrospun nanofibers membranes for air filtration, *Mater. Sci. Eng. C*, **102**, pp. 718–729.

14. Brochot, C., Bahloul, A., Abdolghadr, P. and Haghighat, F. (2019). Performance of mechanical filters used in general ventilation against nanoparticles, *IOP Conf. Ser.: Mater. Sci. Eng.*, **609**, p. 032044.

15. Brouwer, D. H., Lidén, G., Asbach, C., Berges, M. G. M. and van Tongeren, M. (2014). Monitoring and sampling strategy for (manufactured) nano objects, agglomerates and aggregates (NOAA): potential added value of the nanodevice project. In: Vogel, U., Savolainen, K., Wu, Q., van Tongeren, M., Brouwer, D. and Berges, M. (eds.), *Hanbook of Nanosafety*, Chapter 5, Elsevier Inc., pp. 173–206.

16. Burnett, R. T., Pope, C. A., Ezzati, M., Olives, C., Lim, S. S., Mehta, S., Shin, H. H., Singh, G., Hubbell, B., Brauer, M., Anderson, H. R., Smith, K. R., Balmes, J. R., Bruce, N. G., Kan, H., Laden, F., Prüss-Ustün, A., Turner, M. C., Gapstur, S. M., Diver, W. R., Cohen, A. (2014). An integrated risk function for estimating the global burden of disease attributable to ambient fine particulate matter exposure, *Environ. Health Perpect.*, **122**, pp. 397–403.

17. CEB – COVID-19 (2020). Spray com nanopartículas de prata pode ser aliado no combate ao coronavírus. <https://www.cocen.unicamp.br/noticias/id/579/spray-com-nanoparticulas-de-prata-pode-ser-aliado-no-combate-ao-coronavirus>(accessed on July 29, 2020).

18. Chaudhary, J. Tailor, G., Kumar, D. and Joshi, A. (2017). Synthesis and thermal properties of copper nanoparticles, *Asian J. Chem.*, **29**(7), pp. 1492–1494.

19. Chellamani, K. P., Veerasubramanian, D. and Balaji, R. S. V. (2013). Surgical face masks: manufacturing methods and classification. *J. Acad. Ind. Res.*, **2**(6), pp. 320–324.

20. Cheremisinoff, P. N. (1993). *Air Pollution Control and Design for Industry*. Marcel Dekker: United States.

21. Chin, A. W. H., Chu, J. T. S., Perera, M. R. A., Hui, K. P. Y., Yen, H.-L., Chan, M. C. W., et al. (2020). Stability of SARS-CoV-2 in different environmental conditions, *Lancet Microbe*, **1**(1), p. e10.

22. Cho, K. J., Turkevich, L., Miller, M., McKay, R., Grinshpun, S. A., Ha, K.C. and Reponen, T. (2013). Penetration of fiber versus spherical particles through filter media and faceseal leakage of N95filtering facepiece respirators with cyclic flow, *J. Occup. Environ. Hyg.*, **10**, pp. 109–115.

23. Colbeck, I. and Lazaridis, M. (2014). Filtration mechanisms. In: Colbeck, I., Lazaridis, M. (eds.), *Aerosol Science: Technology and Applications*, 1st ed., John Wiley and Sons: United States, pp. 89–118.

24. Das, O., Neisiany, R. E., Capezza, A. J., Hedenqvist, M. S., Försth, M., Xu, Q., Jiang, L., Ji, D. and Ramakrishna, S. (2020). The need for fully bio-based facemasks to counter coronavirus outbreaks: a perspective. *Sci. Total Environ.*, **736**, p. 139611.

25. Dean, J. A. (1999). *Lange's Handbook of Chemistry*, 15th ed. McGraw-Hill: United States.

26. Dullien, A. L. (1989). Aerodynamic capture of particles. In: *Introduction to Industrial Gas Cleaning*. London: Academic Press. pp. 97–121.

27. Ebnesajjab, S. (2009). *Adhesives Technology Handbook*. 2nd ed. William Andrew: United States.

28. Europe Union – EU (2003). Indoor air pollution: new EU research reveals higher risks than previously thought - IP/03/1278, *European Comission*, pp. 1–5.

29. Fitch, E. C. (2010). Filtration mechanics – how filters capture particles. *Machinery Lubrification*.

30. Flagan, R. C. and Seinfeld, J. H. (2012) with Zhongchao, T. (2014). *Air Pollution and Greenhouse Gases: From Basic Concepts to Engineering Applications for Air Emission Control*. Springer: Singapore, p. 95.

31. Gibson, P., Schreuder-Gibson, H. and Rivin, D. (2001). Transport properties of porous membranes based on electrospun nanofiber, *Colloid. Surface. A*, **187–188**, pp. 469–481.

32. Gołofit-Szymczak, M., Stobnicka-Kupiec, A. and Górny, R., L. (2019). Impact of air-conditioning system disinfection on microbial contamination of passenger cars, *Air Qual. Atmos. Health*, **12**, pp. 1127–1135.

33. Grinshpun, S. A. (2010). Biological aerosols. In: Agranovski, I. (ed.), *Aerosols – Science and Technology*. Wiley-VCH: Weinheim, pp. 379–406.

34. Hanage, W. P. (2010). The next pandemic: on the front lines against humankind's gravest dangers, *J. Emerg. Infect. Dis.*, **23**(12), p. 2123.

35. Hang, Q., Welch, J., Park, H., Wu, C. Y., Sigmund, W. and Marijnissen, J. C. M. (2010). Improvement in nanofiber filtration by multiple thin layers of nanofiber mats, *J. Aerosol Sci.*, **41**(2), pp. 230–236.

36. Hinds, C. W. (1998). *Aerosol Technology: Properties, Behaviour, and Measurement of Airborne Particles*, 2nd ed. John Wiley: New York, United States.

37. Hung, C. and Leung, W. W. F. (2011). Filtration of nano-aerosol using nanofiber filter under low Peclet number and transitional flow regime, *Sep. Purif. Technol.*, **79**, pp. 34–42.

38. Hussain, C. M. (2020). *Handbook of Functionalized Nanomaterials for Industrial Applications*, 1st ed. Institute of Technology: Newark, United States.

39. Hyun, J., Lee, S.-G. and Hwang, J. (2017). Application of corona discharge-generated air ions for filtration of aerosolized virus and inactivation of filtered virus, *J. Aerosol Sci.*, **107**, pp. 31–40.

40. International Organization for Standardization (2011). UNE-EN ISO 28439: Workplace atmospheres – Characterization of ultrafine aerosols/nanoaerosols – Determination of the size distribution and number concentration using differential electrical mobility analysing systems, International Organization for Standardization, Geneva, Switzerland.

41. International Organization for Standardization (2013). UNE-EN ISO 29462: Field testing of general ventilation filtration devices and systems for in situ removal efficiency by particle size and resistance to airflow, International Organization for Standardization: Geneva, Switzerland.

42. International Organization for Standardization (2016). UNE-EN ISO 16890: Air filters for general ventilation, International Organization for Standardization: Geneva, Switzerland.

43. Instituto de Pesquisas Tecnológicas (2020). Nanocobre contra vírus e bactérias <https://www.ipt.br/noticia/1632-nanocobre_contra_virus_e_bacterias.htm#.Xx7tT1NEtPo.twitter> (accessed on July 29, 2020).

44. Jo, W.-K. and Lee, J.-H. (2008). Airborne fungal and bacterial levels associatedwith the use of automobile air conditioners or heaters, room air conditioners, and humidifiers, *Arch. Environ. Occup. Health*, **63**(3), pp. 101–107.

45. Johnson, D. F., Druce, J. D., Birch, C. and Grayson, M. L. (2009). A quantitative assessment of the efficacy of surgical and N95 masks to filter influenza virus in patients with acute influenza infection, *Clin. Infect. Dis.*, **49**, pp. 275–277.

46. Jung, J. H., Hwang, G. B., Lee, J. E. and Bae, G. N. (2011). Preparation of airborne Ag/CNT hybrid nanoparticles using an aerosol process and their application to antimicrobial air filtration, *Langmuir*, **27**(16), pp. 10256–10264.

47. Kadam, V. V., Wang, L. and Padhye, R. (2016). Electrospun nanofibre materials to filter air pollutants: a review, *J. Ind. Text.*, **47**(8), pp. 2253–2280.

48. Kampa, M. and Castanas, E. (2008). Human health effects of air pollution, *Environ. Pollut.*, **151**, pp. 362–367.

49. Kelkar, U., Bal, A. M. and Kulkarni, S. (2005). Fungal contamination of air conditioning units in operating theatres in India, *J. Hosp. Infect.*, **60**, pp. 81–84.

50. Kim, H.-J., Han, B., Kim, Y.-J., Oda, T. and Won, H. (2013). Submicrometer particle removal indoors by a novel electrostatic precipitator with high clean air delivery rate, low ozone emissions, and carbon fiber ionizer, *Indoor Air*, **23**(5), pp. 369–378.

51. Kim, K.-H., Kabir, E. and Kabir, S. (2015). A review on the human health impact of airborne particulate matter, *Environ. Int.*, **74**, pp. 136–143.

52. Kirsch, V. A. and Kirsch, A. A. (2010). Deposition of aerosol nanoparticles in model fibrous filters. In: Agranovski, I. (ed.), *Aerosols: Science and Technology*. Wiley-VCH: Weinheim, pp. 283–214.

53. Konda, A., Prakash, A., Moss, G. A., Shcmoldt, M., Grant, G. D. and Guha, S. (2020). Aerosol filtration efficiency of common fabrics used in respiratory cloth masks, *ACS Nano*, **14**, pp. 6339–6347.

54. Kothari, V. K. (2008). *Progress in Textiles: Science and Technology in Technical Textiles Technology, Developments and Applications*, vol. 3, 1st ed. IAFL Publications: India.

55. Koushkbaghi, S., Jafari, P., Rabiei, J., Irani, M. and Aliabadi, M. (2016). Fabrication of PET/PAN/GO/Fe3O4 nanofibrous membrane for the removal of Pb (II) and Cr (VI) ions, *Chem. Eng. J.*, **301**, pp. 42–50.

56. Kravtsov, A., Brünig, H., Zhandarov, S. and Beyreuther, R. (2000). The electret effect in polypropylene fibers treated in a corona discharge, *Adv. Polym. Tech.*, **19**(4), pp. 312–316.

57. Lelieveld, J., Evans, J. S., Fnais, M., Giannadaki, D. and Pozzer, A. (2015). The contribution of outdoor air pollution sources to premature mortality on a global scale, *Nature*, **525**, pp. 367–371.

58. Leung, W. W. F. and Sun, Q. (2020a). Charged PVDF multilayer nanofiber filter in filtering simulated airborne novel coronavirus (COVID-19) using ambient nano-aerosols, *Sep. Purif. Technol.*, **245**, pp. 1–12.

59. Leung, W. W. F. and Sun, Q. (2020b). Electrostatic charged nanofiber filter for filtering airborne novel coronavirus (COVID-19) and nano-aerosols, *Sep. Purif. Technol.*, **250**, pp. 1–17.

60. Li, J., Li, M., Shen, F., Zou, Z., Yao, M. and Wu, C.-Y. (2013). Characterization of biological aerosol exposure risks from automobile air conditioning system, *Environ. Sci. Technol.*, **47**, pp. 10660–10666.

61. Li, X., Wang, C., Huang, X., Zhang, T., Wang, X., Min, M., Wang, L., Huang, H. and Hsiao, B. S. (2018). Anionic surfactant-triggered steiner geometrical poly(vinylidene fluoride) nanofiber/nanonet air filter for efficient particulate matter removal, *ACS Appl. Mater. Interfaces*, **10**, pp. 42891–42904.

62. Li, Z., Kang, W., Zhao, H., Hu, M., Ju, J., Deng, N. and Cheng, B. (2016). Fabrication of a polyvinylidene fluoride tree-like nanofiber web for ultra high performance air filtration, *RSC Adv.*, **6**, p. 91243.

63. Liu, H., Huang, J., Mao, J., Chen, Z., Chen, G. and Lai, Y. (2019). Transparent antibacterial nanofiber air filters with highly efficient moisture resistance for sustainable particulate matter capture. *Science*, **19**, pp. 214–223.

64. Lu, J., Gu, J., Li, K., Xu, C., Su, W., Lai, Z., Zhou, D., Yu, C., Xu, B. and Yang, Z. (2020). COVID-19 outbreak associated with air conditioning in restaurant, Guangzhou, China, 2020, *Emerg. Infect. Dis.*, **26**(7), pp. 1628–1631.

65. Lv, D., Wang, R., Tang, G., Mou, Z., Lei, J., Han, J., Smedt, S. De, Xiong, R. and Huang, C. (2019). Eco-friendly electrospun membranes loaded with visible-light response nano-particles for multifunctional usages: high-efficient air filtration, dye scavenger and bactericide, *ACS Appl. Mater. Interfaces*, **11**(13), pp. 12880–12889.

66. Mao, N. (2017). Nonwoven fabric filters. In: Brown, P. J. and Cox, C. L. (eds.), *Fibrous Filter Media*. Woodhead Publishing, pp. 133–171.

67. Mazumdar, S., Poussou, S. B., Lin, C. H., Isukapalli, S. S., Plesniak, M. W. and Chen, Q. (2011). Impact of scaling and body movement on contaminant transport in airliner cabins, *Atmos. Environ.*, **45**(33), pp. 6019–6028.

68. Meng, X., Zhang, Y., Yang, K.-Q., Yang, Y.-K. and Zhou, X.-L. (2016). Potential harmful effects of $PM_{2.5}$ on occurrence and progression of acute coronary syndrome: epidemiology, mechanisms, and prevention measures, *Int. J. Environ. Res. Public Health*, **13**, p. 748.

69. Morawska, L. and Cao, J. (2020). Airborne transmission of SARS-CoV-2: the world should face the reality, *Environ. Int.*, **139**, p. 105730.

70. Morawska, L., Johnson, G. R., Ristovski, Z. D., Hargreaves, M., Mengersen, K., Corbett, S., Chao, C. Y. H., Li, Y. and Katoshevski, D. (2009). Size distribution and sites of origin of droplets expelled from

the human respiratory tract during expiratory activities, *J. Aerosol Sci.*, **40**(3), pp. 256–269.

71. Neeltje, V. D., Morris, D. H., Holbrook, M. G., Gamble, A., Williamson, B. N., Tamin, A., Harcourt, N. J., Thornburg, J. N., Gerber, S. I., Lloyd-Smith, J. O., Wit, E. de., Munster, V. J. (2020). Aerosol and surface stability of SARS-CoV-2 as compared with SARS-CoV-1, *N. Engl.*, **382**, pp. 1564–1567.

72. Nuvolone, D., Petri, D. and Voller, F. (2018). The effects of ozone on human health, *Environ. Sci. Pollut. Res.*, **25**, pp. 8074–8088.

73. Park, D. H., Joe, Y. H., Piri, A., An, S. and Hwang, J. (2020). Determination of air filter anti-viral efficiency against an airborne infectious virus, *J. Hazard. Mater.*, **396**, p. 122640.

74. Park, J. H., Yoon, K. Y. and Hwang, J. H. (2011). Removal of submicron particles using a carbon fiber ionizer-assisted medium airfilter in a heating, ventilation, and air-conditioning (HVAC) system, *Build. Environ.*, **46**, pp. 1699–1708.

75. Perumalraj, R. (2016). Characterization of electrostatic discharge properties of woven fabrics, *J. Text. Eng.*, **6**, p. 235.

76. Power, M. C., Weisskopf, M. G., Alexeeff, S. E., Coull, B. A., Spiro, III, A, and Schwartz, J. (2011). Traffic-related air pollution and cognitive function in a cohort of older men, *Environ. Health Perspect.*, **119**, pp. 682–687.

77. Prezekop, R. and Gradon, L. (2008). Deposition and filtration of nanoparticles in the composites of nano- and microsized fibers, *Aerosol Sci. Tech.*, **42**(6), pp. 483–493.

78. Purchas, D. B. and Sutherland, K. (2002). *Handbook of Filter Media*. Elsevier Science & Technology Books.

79. Purwar, R., Goutham, K. S. and Srivastava, C. M. (2016). Electrospun sericin/PVA/clay nanofibrous mats for antimicrobial air filtration mask, *Fibers Polym.*, **17**(8), pp. 1206–1216.

80. Pyankov, O., Agranovski, I., Huang, R. and Mullins, B. (2008). Removal of biological aerosols by oil coated filters, *Clean-Soil Air Water*, **36**(7), pp. 609–614.

81. Qian, Y., Willeke, K., Grinshpun, S. A., Donnelly, J. and Coffey, C. C. (1998). Performance of N95 respirators: filtration efficiency for airborne microbial and inert particles, *Am. Ind. Hyg. Assoc.*, **59**(2), pp. 128–132.

82. Rahimi, M. and Mokhtari, J. (2018). Modeling and optimization of waterproof-breathable thermo-regulating core-shell nanofiber/net structured membrane for protective clothing applications, *Polym. Eng. Sci.*, **58**(10), pp. 1756–1765.

83. Ramyadevi, J., Jeyasubramanian, K., Marikani, A., Rajakumar, G. and Rahuman, A. A. (2012). Synthesis and antimicrobial activity of copper nanoparticles, *Mater. Lett.*, **71**, pp. 114–116.

84. Riehle, C. (1997). Electrostatic precipitation. In: Seville, J. P. K. (ed.), *Gas Cleaning in Demanding Applications*. Blackie Academic & Professional, London, pp. 193–228.

85. Robinson, M. C. and Hollis Hallett, A. C. (1966). The static dielectric constant of NaCl, KCl, and KBr at temperatures between 4.2°K and 300°K, *Can. J. Phys.*, **44**(10), pp. 2211–2230.

86. Rohit, A., Rajasekaran, S., Karunasagar, I. and Karunasagar, I. (2020). Fate of respiratory droplets in tropical vs temperate environments and implications for SARS-CoV-2 transmission, *Med. Hypotheses*, **144**, p. 109958.

87. Rosa, P. F., Aguiar, M. L. and Bernardo, A. (2017). Modification of cotton fabrics with silver nanoparticles for use in conditioner air to minimize the bioaerosol concentration in indoor environments, *Water Air Soil Pollut.*, **228**, p. 244.

88. SC INOVA (2020). Nanotecnologia versus COVID-19: empresa de SC cria produto que elimina vírus de roupas e superfícies. <https://scinova.com.br/nanotecnologia-versus-covid-19-empresa-de-sc-cria-produto-que-elimina-virus-de-roupas-e-superficies/> (acessed on July 29, 2020).

89. Scheller, C., Krebs, F., Minkner, R., Astner, I., Gil-Moles, M. and Wätzig, H. (2020). Physicochemical properties of SARS-CoV-2 for drug targeting, virus inactivation and attenuation, vaccine formulation and quality control, *Electrophoresis*, **41**(13–14), pp. 1137–1151.

90. Schraufnagel, D. E., Balmes, J. R., Cowl, C. T., De Matteis, S., Jung, S.-H., Mortimer, K., Perez-Padilla, R., Rice, M. B., Riojas-Rodriguez, H., Sood, A., Thurston, G. D., To, T., Vanker, A. and Wuebbles, D. J. (2019). Air pollution and noncommunicable diseases: a review by the forum of international respiratory societies' environmental committee, part 2: air pollution and organ systems, *Chest*, **155**, pp. 417–426.

91. Setti, L., Passarini, F., De Gennaro, G., Barbieri, P., Perrone, M. G., Borelli, M., Palmisani, J., Di Gilio, A., Piscitelli, P. and Miani, A. (2020). Airborne transmission route of COVID-19: why 2 meters/6 feet of inter-personal distance could not be enough, *Int. J. Environ. Res. Public Health*, **17**(8), p. 2932.

92. Shi, L., Zhuang, X., Tao, X., Cheng, B. and Kang, W. (2013). Solution blowing nylon 6 nanofiber mats for air filtration, *Fibers Polym.*, **14**(9), pp. 1485–1490.

93. Stadnytskyi, V., Bax, C. E., Bax, A. and Anfinrud, P. (2020). The airborne lifetime of small speech droplets and their potential importance in SARS-CoV-2 transmission, *PNAS*, **117**(22), pp. 11875–11877.

94. Strauss, W. (1975). The aerodynamic capture of particles. In: *Industrial Gas Cleaning*, 2nd ed. London: Pergamon Press, pp. 277–313.

95. Sung, A. D., Sung, J. A. M., Thomas, S., Hyslop, T., Gasparetto, C., Long, G., Rizzieri, D., Sullivan, K. M., Corbet, K., Broadwater, G., Chao, N. J. and Horwitz, M. E. (2016). Universal mask usage for reduction of respiratory viral infections after stem cell transplant: a prospective trial, *Clin. Infect. Dis.*, **63**, pp. 999–1006.

96. Sunyer, J., Esnaola, M., Alvarez-Pedrerol, M., Forns, J., Rivas, I., López-Vicente, M., Suades-González, E., Foraster, M., Garcia-Esteban, R., Basagaña, X., Viana, M., Cirach, M., Moreno, T., Alastuey, A., Sebastian-Galles, N., Nieuwenhuijsen, M. and Querol, X. (2015). Association between traffic-related air pollution in schools and cognitive development in primary school children: a prospective cohort study, *PLoS Med.*, **12**(3), p. e1001792.

97. Sutherland, K. and Chase, G. (2008). *Filters and Filtration Handbook*, 5th ed. Elsevier.

98. Tan, Z. (2014). *Air Pollution and Greenhouse Gases, Green Energy and Technology*. Springer: Singapore.

99. Tremiliosi, G. C., Simoes, L. G. P., Minozzi, D. T., Renato, I., Vilela, D. C. B., Durigon, E. L., Machado, R. R. G., Medina, D. S., Ribeiro, L. K., Rosa, I. L. V., Assis, M., Andrés, J., Longo, E., Freitas Jr., L. H. (2020). Ag nanoparticles-based antimicrobial polycotton fabrics to prevent the transmission and spread of SARS-CoV-2, doi:10.1101/2020.06.26.152520.

100. Wang, N., Cai, M., Yang, X. and Yang, Y. (2018). Electret nanofibrous membrane with enhanced filtration performance and wearing comfortability for face mask, *J. Colloid Interface Sci.*, **530**, pp. 695–703.

101. Waring, M. S., Siegel, J. A. and Corsi, R. L. (2008). Ultrafine particle removal and generation by portable air cleaners, *Atmos. Environ.*, **42**(20), pp. 5003–5014.

102. Warnes, S. L., Little, Z. R. and Keevil, C. W. (2015). Human coronavirus 229E remains infectious on common touch surface materials, *MBio*, **6**(6), doi:10.1128/mBio.01697-15.

103. Weaver, L., Noyce, J. O., Michels, H. T. and Keevil, C. W. (2010). Potential action of copper surfaces on meticillin-resistant *Staphylococcus aureus*, *J. Appl. Microbiol.*, **109**(6), pp. 2200–2205.

104. Wiedensohler, A. (1988). An approximation of the bipolar charge distribution for particles in the submicron size range, *J. Aerosol Sci.*, **19**(3), pp. 387–389.

105. World Health Organization (2005). WHO air quality guidelines for particulate matter, ozone, nitrogen dioxide and sulfur dioxide. Global update 2005 - Summary of risk assessment. Retrieved from: <http://www.who.int/phe/health_topics/outdoorair/outdoorair_aqg/en/> (accessed on July 20, 2020).

106. World Health Organization (2010). WHO guidelines for indoor air quality: Selected pollutants. World Health Organization: Denmark.

107. World Health Organization (2020a). Air pollution. Available from: <https://www.who.int/health-topics/air-pollution#tab=tab_1> (accessed on July 29, 2020).

108. World Health Organization (2020b). Q&A: How is COVID-19 transmitted? Available from: <https://www.who.int/emergencies/diseases/novel-coronavirus-2019/question-and-answers-hub/q-a-detail/q-a-how-is-covid-19-transmitted?gclid=CjwKCAjw0_T4BRBlEiwAwoEiAUBRaneBpJ2mj-dS_UUs9bo0RzjiclCpOsB6cuu8Nf6h49Us86Df5hoCoQ8QAvD_BwE> (accessed on July 29, 2020).

109. World Health Organization (2020c). Coronavirus disease (COVID-19) – Situation Report – 190. Available from: <https://www.who.int/docs/default-source/coronaviruse/situation-reports/20200728-covid-19-sitrep-190.pdf?sfvrsn=fec17314_2 (accessed on July 28, 2020).

110. Yu, L., Peel, G. K., Cheema, F. H., Lawrence, W. S., Bukreyeva, N., Jinks, C. W., Peel, J. E., Peterson, J. W., Paessler, S., Hourani, M. and Ren, Z. (2020). Catching and killing of airborne SARS-CoV-2 to control spread of COVID-19 by a heated air disinfection system, *Mater. Today Phys.*, **15**, p. 100249.

111. Zhang, Q., Honko, A., Zhou, J., Gong, H., Downs, S. N., Vasquez, J. H., Fang, R. H., Gao, W., Griffiths, A. and Zhang, L. (2020). Cellular nanosponges inhibit SARS-CoV-2 infectivity, *Nano Lett.*, **20**(7), pp. 5570–5574.

112. Zhang, X., Ji, Z., Yue, Y., Liu, H. and Wang, J. (2020). Infection risk assessment of COVID-19 through aerosol transmission: a case study of south china seafood market, *Environ. Sci. Technol.* (in press), doi:10.1021/acs.est.0c02895.

113. Zhongchao, T. (2014). Separation of particles from a gas. In: *Air Pollution and Greenhouse Gases: From Basic Concepts to Engineering*

Applications for Air Emission Control. Springer: Singapore, pp. 151–226.

114. Zhou, S. S., Lukula, S., Chiossone, C., Nims, R. W., Suchmann, D. B. and Ijaz, M. K. (2018). Assessment of a respiratory mask for capturing air pollutants and pathogens including human influenza and rhinoviruses, *J. Thorac. Dis.*, **10**(3), pp. 2059–2069.

115. Zhu, N., Zhang, D., Wang, W., Li, X., Yang, B., Song, J., Zhao, X., Huang, B., Shi, W., Lu, R., Niu, P., Zhan, F., Ma, X., Wang, D., Xu, W., Wu, G., Gao, G. F. and Tan, W. (2019). A novel coronavirus from patients with pneumonia in China, 2019, *N. Eng. J. Med.*, **382**, pp. 727–733.

Index

Milton Keynes UK
Ingram Content Group UK Ltd.
UKHW022113220124
436509UK00001B/1